Guided M

CW00969214

For Health & Wellbeing

Dan Jones

First Edition 2015

Published By Dan Jones

ISBN: 978-1507815168

Cover Image: © Bakharev | Dreamstime.com

Contents

Introduction

Meditation has a long history; meditation is a fundamental part of most major religions and spiritual practices. In recent year's mindfulness meditation and loving kindness meditations especially have received significant interest from the scientific community for the health and wellbeing benefits that they bring. Mindfulness meditation is now often incorporated into Cognitive Behavioural Therapy and there is even Mindfulness-Based Cognitive Behavioural Therapy and Mindfulness-Based Stress Reduction (MBSR) becoming popular as recognised forms of treatment.

Mindfulness meditation focuses on being in the moment, on being like a person sitting in a park gazing up at the clouds and calmly just watching those clouds pass by. Some of the clouds are dark and stormy, others are white and fluffy, yet the person just sits in the park watching those clouds pass acknowledging that they are there, but not being drawn into giving judgements about the clouds they are watching.

Mindfulness meditation has tremendous value as a therapeutic tool; there are many situations that require being able to be just in the moment, not focusing on the negatives of the past, or worrying about what might be in the future. Often these thinking styles can cloud our judgement leading to poor decision making and experiencing negative feelings here in the present. If a person judges that they have always failed previously they may judge that they are a failure and why bother trying now. Or if someone worries that a talk they need to give will go wrong, then they are less likely to prepare properly for the talk and so less likely to be confident giving the talk or do well giving the talk.

What mindfulness meditation can teach is the ability to use guided attachment. Some practitioners talk about non-attachment and the importance of becoming non-attached to things in life. What I feel is healthier is to learn to guide your attachments, so that you can attach to what is important moment by moment. Attachment is required for certain things in life and unless you hope to become a hermit living a solitary life where you don't want to be weighed down by attachments and desires, and want to be able to just be in the moment wherever you are then there will be some things that you will want to be attached to. To form and maintain healthy relationships we need attachment, to achieve success in life we need attachment, and to learn effectively we need attachment. So many of the meditations in this book focus on guided attachment, on ensuring that your focus is attached to what is important, and not attached to what isn't important. Many of the meditations in this book are goal-oriented meditations, so they are meditations with purpose that help focus your attention on ideas, thoughts and mentally rehearsing changes that can be helpful in achieving success.

Loving kindness meditation focuses on compassion, on compassion for others, and for yourself, on love for others and yourself including a desire for other beings and yourself to have what is needed for happiness, on sympathetic joy, which is deriving happiness, pleasure and joy from others experiencing happiness and joy, and an acceptance that underneath the surface reality of chaos and apparent difference all beings are the same.

Loving kindness meditation can help us to feel good about ourselves and others. Focusing on gratitude, on being grateful for whom we are, what we have, and for what our experiences are helps to lift depression and increase feelings of wellbeing as we see a more positive side to life. For example in the story that follows I will share a tale from my life with you. The outcome of the tale is that I was thinking about how lucky I was that I was hit by a truck, how lucky I was that it was early in the morning, how lucky I was with my injuries, how lucky I was that I was able to learn more about myself and my meditation skills, how lucky I was that I had new opportunities open up to me that weren't there before I got ran over.

The meditations in this book are all guided meditations and different to most other guided meditations. Often guided meditations are just guided stories. These meditations are based on various principles of meditation and are using meditation therapeutically. Part of the difference between these meditations and other meditations are that they incorporate mental rehearsal and therapeutic principles as well as meditation principles.

When I first started to think about writing this book I knew I would be taking a risk, because I would be presenting meditations that are likely to appear unfamiliar to people, they use principles of meditation to create something therapeutic and effective, but something that appears different to most meditations people are used to.

This is something that occurs in therapy, where an experienced therapist can take a standard therapeutic technique, identify the principles underlying the technique and its effectiveness, and then create variations of the technique that look nothing like the original technique but are equally as effective. This is often what sets an experienced therapist apart from a newly trained therapist. The experienced therapist can tailor the technique to the client, rather than trying to fit all clients to the one technique.

All meditations fall into either mindfulness-based where the idea is to have awareness but not attachment, and if attention becomes focused in on part of the experience then recognising this before moving the attention away again to just observing, and concentration-based where the idea is to focus attention on one thing and hold it there, and if it strays then bring it back to that one focus point.

Guided meditations can involve stories as teaching tales that stimulate the mind to focus on specific mental patterns, or to recognise specific situations, they can involve guided imagery or relaxing imagery as a way of focusing the mind inwardly to separate from external reality and from what the meditator has been focusing on prior to the meditation towards what will be more helpful for them to focus on, the initial guided imagery or relaxation stage can act as a transition stage between one state and another.

Guided meditations can involve mental rehearsal. Many guided meditations are kept just metaphorical leaving it to the instinctive part of the meditators mind to work out the meaning and what it is supposed to do. From years of experience I have found that it is helpful to guide someone into a meditative state where they are focused on what is important to move forward from their problem, and then whilst they are focused have them mentally rehearse what life will be like doing things in this new and improved way.

There is significant research around the positive benefits of mental rehearsal where the mind can't tell the difference between real and vividly imagined. In one study people were split into two groups, one group practiced throwing a basketball into a basketball hoop, the other group handled the ball to know what it felt like and then mentally rehearsed successfully throwing a basketball into a basketball hoop repeatedly. Those that mentally rehearsed did better than those that practiced for real – why? Because those that practiced for real made plenty of mistakes as well as successful shots, whereas those that mentally rehearsed only practiced being successful, so taught their mind and body only what it needed to do, not multiple ways of doing things right and wrong. The ideal situation is to mix both, practice for real, and rehearse for success.

How do you use these meditations?

These meditations are designed to be self-recorded as audio tracks or read to the person or people that will be experiencing the meditation, they are great for reading to individuals and for use when doing group guided meditations. There is no single way they should be recorded. The best advice on how to record the personal meditation tracks is to record them how you would like them to be spoken to you. Ideally you will want the track to be relaxing to listen to, you could get a friend to record tracks for you if you have a friend with a voice you think would be ideal to help you relax. As you read the meditation you will be recording you can practice how you would like the rhythm of the reading to happen, and how you would like pauses. Some people like long pauses to help them become absorbed, others prefer shorter pauses.

An interesting phenomenon is how silence deepens the experience. Often having too much silence at the beginning of a meditation makes the meditation seem too slow for many people, but once people have started to go with the experience then silence takes on a whole new meaning, when the voice stops people usually just drift deeper and deeper into the experience. After a period of time people often find their inner voice goes quiet as they follow along to what is being said, so when the person talking is quiet and the individual's inner voice is quiet the person suddenly experiences a state of nothingness where there is no talking inside or outside, and no thoughts going through the mind, so they have nothing to use to measure time. Sometimes this can feel like a shock to the person meditating when they suddenly realise that they have been sitting in silence for a period of time, and are unable to tell how long they have been in silence for and suddenly realise their mind has been blank for many minutes.

Often audio meditations are more effective when listened to through headphones. Wearing headphones makes the experience more absorbing.

Meditations aren't something you can listen to once and then expect changes to be instant, for the meditation to work the meditator needs to listen regularly, ideally daily so that the meditation can begin to work. The meditator is learning through regular meditation. In the same way that you wouldn't take one pill and expect it to solve a medical problem, you would take the required dose every day until you are better, or you wouldn't expect to sit at a piano and play it perfectly the first go, you would practice daily and gradually get better each day.

Each meditation will be teaching the meditator something about what to focus on and attach to and what not to attach to as a way of overcoming problems. There is no set length meditation should be, but what people often find is that their experience of an ideal length of time meditating fits with what has come from scientific research on ultradian rhythms. Ultradian rhythms are biological rhythms of less than 24 hours. We also have a circadian rhythm which is about 25 hours long which is the familiar sleep/awake cycle we follow, and we have infradian rhythms, these are rhythms of greater than 24 hours, like the menstrual cycle.

Ultradian rhythms include the rhythm of our heart, breathing, and cell division. The best known ultradian rhythm is the basic rest and activity cycle (BRAC). This is a 90-120 minute cycle of being more alert and more inwardly focused. The cycle continues all day every day through our waking and sleeping, it rises over a period of about 40 minutes to a peak state of alertness where you are likely to feel most productive and awake, holding that peak for perhaps 15-20 minutes before heading down towards a trough of inner focus which lasts for about 15-20 minutes. This inner focus stage is the stage where people most frequently want to take a break when they are at work, it is the period when you daydream most, and when you struggle to keep your focus on tasks you are doing. This is the point many people take stimulants to try to 'snap out of it'.

Imagine a day where you wake up at 7.30 am for work, you leave for work about 8.30 am and arrive at work about 9am. Often the first thing people want is to take a break even though they have just arrived at work, so people often grab a drink and take 15-20 minutes to properly settle into work. Some people are aware they do this and so wake up slightly earlier, set off to work slightly earlier and take a break just before they start work. About 90-120 minutes later they feel a need to take a break again about 11am, then again about 1pm and 3pm before finally leaving work about 5pm just when they are feeling like it should be time to go home. Around 2-3pm is normally the time our BRAC is at its lowest, and also is the lowest daytime point of our circadian rhythm, and if we have eaten a large lunch this can trigger the release of hormones designed to relax us further, making a siesta a very good idea at this point. Often people aim to have dinner about 7pm which fits with the next ultradian dip, and perhaps a bath or something relaxing about 9pm, before settling to bed about 10:30pm-11pm.

This pattern above is when things are working most ideal. If someone does shift work or works long hours they may not be able to be this structured. Generally people that feel alert most of the day, that feel like they function well through the day and then sleep well at night are likely to have a pattern fairly close to this, they may start work earlier or later and so have the pattern shifted, but they are likely to follow this 90-120 minute cycle.

This cycle crops up in other areas, like films or shows usually being 90-120 minutes long, often if a film or a show is longer than this people start to get restless and want to take a break. And people not being able to have a rhythm close to this regular 90-120 minute cycle are more prone to having mood problems or compensatory problems, like addictions that stimulate like smoking or drinking coffee to push through the troughs, or addictions to depressants like alcohol to come down from an alert peak to a trough to help them to relax.

As the basic rest and activity cycle happens all day every day, if you meditate for longer than about twenty minutes your mind and body may be approaching a peak of alertness, whilst you are trying to remain relaxed. When people are left to meditate for whatever time period feels about right they normally do so for around 15-20 minutes, and the best time for this is at a time when your mind is naturally beginning to wander and it feels like you need to take a break and relax. These meditations in this book are about 15 minutes long when read in a calm, slow relaxing voice to be ideal for helping you get the benefits of the meditation without becoming too drowsy or restless. Many of the meditations involve around 8-10 minutes of speech before allowing for the meditation to then continue on in silence for whatever duration is right for you. Often people like to have about 5-10 minutes of silence. This can either be left with the end of the meditation being just silence and the listener will reorient from the meditation once they are ready, or the person talking through the meditation can leave a 5-10 minute pause and then start talking again to bring the person out of the experience.

Often if someone falls asleep meditating it is because they are sleep deprived and so their mind took the opportunity when the person was relaxing to have them sleep in that time to catch up on the sleep they need rather than taking that time to follow the meditation. If you do fall asleep you may feel drowsy on awakening depending how long you have slept for and what stage of sleep you have woken from. If this happens that is alright, you can always listen to the meditation again, if you need the sleep and this helps you get that needed sleep then the meditation may not be achieving what you had hoped for it to achieve, but it will still be helpful to you. If this continues for a prolonged period then it may be worth thinking about what time of the day you choose to meditate, perhaps there is a different time of the day when you are naturally less tired.

My Story

At 6am on the morning of 17th January 2005 I was cycling nine miles to the children's home I had helped to set up. It was a cold and dark morning. Generally I enjoy cycling in these conditions; most of the journey doesn't have street lights so when the sky was clear I was able to look up and enjoy the moon and stars. There is also very little traffic on the roads at this time of the morning.

This specific morning things didn't go as well as usual. I had made it about eight miles into my journey when I reached a roundabout. As I was cycling around the roundabout I could see a truck heading towards the roundabout on the road I was just about to pass across. From the speed the truck was going as it approached the give way lines I could see that it wasn't going to stop. In my mind I was thinking that I wasn't going to be able to stop before crossing the path of the truck, so I was going to have to try to cycle faster to get out the way of the truck before it reached me.

If the truck was driving in the correct lane then I might have managed this, but the truck was driving straight down the centre of the road. The truck struck the side of my bike launching my bike and myself out into the road, I landed in the middle of the road in a seated position, and my bike landed some distance away behind me.

When this incident happened I felt very lucky. I had been cycling wearing ordinary clothing, I was wearing jeans, a black waterproof jacket, steel toecap sand coloured boots and no cycle helmet. When I looked at my boots I could see marks where the truck had hit my left foot. The steel toecap on the boot had protected my foot and the boot had probably protected my ankle from the impact.

Despite not wearing a cycle helmet I didn't sustain any injuries to my head because of being hit by a truck rather than a car. The front of the truck was about as high as my whole bike, so when I was hit I didn't land on the bonnet of the vehicle and hit my unprotected head on the windscreen, instead I was pushed out into the road away from the truck. Because of how I was pushed I came off my bike and struck the road with my right elbow, apart from a few grazes my right elbow was the only part of me that was injured.

Because I was cycling very early in the morning there was very little traffic around so I didn't end up under the wheels of any other cars on the road and help got to me quickly to get me to hospital. When I was hit I was surprised that I didn't feel any pain, I continued to feel no pain while I was on the road waiting to be helped up. Initially I thought maybe I hadn't been injured until I tried to get up. I tried to move my right arm to lean on my right hand to stand and all I heard was a grinding sound. I looked at my right hand and tried to move it again, and again I heard grinding, but saw no movement.

I picked up my right hand with my left hand and held it across my body, but as I was holding my hand I couldn't use either hand to help me stand up and move out of the road. Someone helpful had called the ambulance service and had been advised not to move me. I wouldn't have minded except that there was still traffic heading round the roundabout, and I wasn't keen on being run over because I was sat in the middle of the road.

The helpful lady was talking to the operator saying that I was saying I wanted to be moved, and was being told not to move me. I was aware that this was supposed to be for my benefit, because I had just been involved in an accident so I could have damage that would be made worse by moving me, but from my perspective if I stayed sat in the middle of the road there was a chance I could get hit by a car and seriously injured, and given I had already been seriously injured I wasn't keen on getting seriously injured a second time in the space of five minutes.

After a few minutes of negotiating I managed to convince the helpful woman and the operator she was talking with that it was safer to help me stand and move me to the curb than to leave me in the middle of the road. Unfortunately the woman wasn't strong enough to help me up, luckily though the ambulance arrived at this point and two of the ambulance crew came over to help. They grabbed hold of either side of my trousers and in one quick movement lifted me uncomfortably to my feet and helped me to the ambulance.

It was lighter in the ambulance than it had been out on the road, I was able to see blood dripping from the fingers of my right hand and could see my coat looked shredded at the elbow and there appeared to be a lot of blood. One of the ambulance crew told me he was going to have to cut the ring off my finger on my right hand as my hand was beginning to swell, I tried to move my hand and fingers again but nothing happened all I could hear was a grinding, crunching sound like standing on crisps. I still didn't have any pain, although I was feeling light-headed and wanted to close my eyes and sleep. Although I don't now believe I was at risk of dying, at the time I had a thought that if I closed my eyes to sleep I may never open them again, so I kept my eyes open and kept talking with the ambulance crew all the way to hospital.

At the hospital I had relaxed more, it was now about thirty minutes since I had been hit by the truck. I was now thinking I want my loved ones to know what has happened and where I am, and I want the children's home informed because they would have been expecting me to arrive and are likely to be wondering where I have got to.

Something that is interesting about pain is that it can be very subjective, so all this time I had been focusing on different aspects of the situation, and avoiding focusing on the pain. I hadn't been saying to myself 'I am hurt', or 'this hurts'. I had been focusing on what needs to happen, from focusing on getting out of the road to be safe from harm, to talking with the ambulance crew in the ambulance about wanting people informed once we get to hospital that I have been involved in an accident and letting them know where I am. Then at the hospital I wanted it confirmed that people had been informed.

I never once asked what my injuries were; I never once focused on what injuries I thought I had. I had tried to do things without success, like trying to move my hand and arm, and I had seen things like the blood that could have made me panic. I had even started to have the thought that I could die, but chose to focus externally on talking with the ambulance crew rather than panicking. I did choose not to do the behaviour I imagined was linked to whether I would die or not, and as I mentioned I now don't think I was really at risk of dying, and if I had asked the ambulance crew directly I would probably have had this confirmed. But my mind gave me the thought and I decided not to worry about it, but also not to do the behaviour I had associated with my thoughts, and decided the best thing to do was to focus externally on talking.

At the hospital a Doctor looked at my right arm, I tried not to see the injuries; I was still not in pain. He took photographs and said that there was a lot of damage. He asked if I wanted to see the photographs. I told him that I didn't because if I saw them it would make my right arm and the injuries real and I felt that this would make me aware of the pain.

Back in 2001 I had completed training in Zen Meditation, Healing Meditation and Tibetan Buddhist Meditation. I spent much of my childhood doing meditation without realising that that was what I was doing. So once I learnt about meditation and discovered I had been doing it for years without realising it I felt I needed to undertake training to learn more about what meditation was and how to do it, and what the benefits of meditation are.

Now this training was coming in handy. I was able to focus my attention on what was immediately important, so I was in control of my attention rather than my attention being in control of me.

By focusing outside of my body and mind I was able to go through the experience this far without needing to have any painkillers and without being distressed. After having my arm looked at I went into surgery for about eight hours to have my arm pieced back together. There were ten breaks in my elbow, it was an open fracture and I had some bone missing that was obviously left behind at the scene of the accident. I needed to have metal pins, plates and screws put into my arm to hold everything together and when I came out of the operation I had my right arm in a very large and thick plaster cast and my left arm had a morphine drip going into it.

I didn't actually see my right arm again for a couple of months when I eventually was allowed to have the cast taken off and the metal staples removed (which again I was told would be painful, so I focused all of my attention on the wall counting how many squares I could see so that I wouldn't be paying attention to what was taking place with my arm).

After my operation I was in hospital for about a week. The morphine drip was a self-administer drip. If I was feeling any pain I was able to push a button to give myself more morphine. I was also being given high doses of Ibuprofen, Codeine and Paracetamol. It is interesting how people naturally like to take the easiest option. For the first few days in hospital I would press the morphine button every time I felt my arm hurt because this was a quick and easy solution to numb the pain. But as time went on I began to get annoyed with the morphine. It seemed to make my mouth move at a different speed to my internal dialogue. I would think of something I wanted to say, and then when I would try to say it, it was as if my mouth went into slow motion. I found that I really struggled to talk properly. Eventually I asked a nurse when I can come off the morphine drip and was told that if I don't self-administer for 24 hours then they will assume I don't need it, and it will be removed.

This motivated me enough to stop being lazy, and instead use the skills I have to address the pain without the aid of drugs. I then began to imagine my arm wasn't a part of me. I focused externally on what was going on, on others on the ward, on visitors, and when it was quiet and lights were out I found somewhere pleasant to go in my mind. After 24 hours I had the morphine drip removed. The Doctors told me I still had to take the other medication, and nurses would come around every few hours day and night to give it to me whether I wanted it or not, but at least I was off the morphine.

When I was discharged I was given high doses of Codeine, Paracetamol and Ibuprofen as well as a bottle of morphine to take. As soon as I left the hospital and was in control of what medication I was taking I chose not to take any of it, and instead managed the pain in my arm using meditation skills I had learnt over the years. Once my arm was fully out of a cast I had lots of pain from my arm being inactive for such a long time. My muscles had wasted and my arm was very weak. Physiotherapy proved to be a painful experience, and I have had ongoing pain ever since as my bones grind every time I move my elbow. This has allowed me to regularly practice and use techniques to reduce and stop the pain. At times, like during physiotherapy I didn't want to have my arm totally numb or not focus on it because it was important that I push myself as far as was safe to do so in the physiotherapy, but not overdo it to the point where I may cause further injuries. So I focused on having sensations but not pain, it is like the difference between analgesia and anaesthesia, analgesia is the removal of pain, but not of sensations and feelings, whereas anaesthesia creates numbness removing the pain, sensations and feelings.

So why have I just taken the time to tell you all this about one significant event in my life?

As a child I grow up in a home where almost anything I did or didn't do resulted in being physically chastised. When eating food I would be hit for eating too fast, so I would slow down, then I would be hit for eating too slow, so I would speed up a little, then I would be hit for 'trying to take the piss'. So I used to take myself out into the woods around the house I lived in and would find a tree to sit in where I would stay for hours at a time.

In the tree I would close my eyes and listen, focusing on the sounds of birds, the sound of the wind as it rustled leaves and blew through the trees, sounds of other animals. I would try to focus my attention on individual birds or sounds and try to work out exactly where the sound was coming from, trying to identify the distance and direction. I would try to work out how many different individual sounds I could hear, and would spend hours relaxing and keeping my mind clear and feeling content and peaceful being just in the moment, not letting thoughts of what has happened or what might happen into my mind.

Until I was hit by a truck I had never had to 'try' to use my meditation skills. I had been using a mindfulness approach for years long before I knew that was what I had been doing. So as an adult I had already learnt to do this instinctively and so didn't have to try to do it, it just happened. This meant that I could be in situations where people were threatening violence and I would naturally remain calm, I could be in job interviews and would be calm and relaxed (although in one situation I was told that I didn't get a job because I appeared too calm, and the interviewers felt this meant I didn't want the job enough, so even if you are calm it is worth having a little nervousness there), and I could be in emergency situations and would be calm and focused.

What I hadn't encountered was having to actively use these skills in situations where I was in pain. This was a whole new learning for me. It is easy to meditate in a calm and peaceful place with no disturbances and no problems or stresses. What is more challenging is being able to translate those learnings to the real world to see if these techniques work when you actually need them.

It is like being on holiday where you can relax, you don't think about bills you need to pay, or work you need to be doing, for that one week you are in a different reality. During the holiday you feel calm and relaxed and refreshed, yet once you are back home and you open all the bills that have arrived whilst you were away, and you work out how much you have just spent, and you check your work emails in anticipation of being back in work the next day and see you have so much work to catch up on, and now you feel all stressed again, it is much harder to maintain that peace and calm at home than it is on holiday.

As a child sitting in a tree it was easy to remain peaceful and calm, I had nothing else in that moment to worry about and I did it so much that I began to naturally be able to be in the moment. I wasn't surprised that I was able to apply these skills instinctively when I got ran over, it was a crisis and so I naturally went into being in the moment and dealing with the crisis. What surprised me was being able to learn how to manage pain and get myself into that state of mind where I was in the moment and just being mindful when I wasn't in a crisis or any emergency.

Initially my response was the same as most people's response; it was to take the drugs to stop the pain. It didn't even cross my mind initially to help myself because the drugs were helping me. This one incident taught me to trust the instinctive part of me, and trust what it has learnt over my lifetime, and that it can apply what it has learnt if I get out of its way consciously. The incident taught me what works and what doesn't work for me, and the extent that meditation can help reduce anxiety, reduce pain, create calm, and help focus and find answers.

Since 2001 I have been working with people using various guided meditation and mindfulness techniques to help others to overcome a wide variety of problems from insomnia to anxiety and weight loss. It is a common saying that to truly know how to help someone you need to know and understand where they are coming from, and those that are often best at this are people that have had the problem they are helping with. I know that I used to think about some things very differently prior to being hit by a truck. Since being hit by a truck I have used mindfulness and guided meditation on myself to help myself with pain, anxiety including post-traumatic stress disorder (PTSD), self-belief, stress, noticing life's opportunities, insomnia and more, and in being able to be successful with myself I have learnt more about what works to be successful with others.

Guided Meditations

It is best to create and listen to just one meditation at a time. If you try to work on too many problems or issues at once it makes it more difficult to achieve success with any one of those issues.

Some people may be able to follow the meditation by slowly reading and imagining in their mind as they read, others may be able to read and memorise the meditation, or the gist of the meditation, but most people will benefit most from audio recording the meditation and listening to the recording daily until changes begin to happen. It is alright to alter some of the wording so that the recording flows naturally for you as an individual, for most people changes are likely to be noticeable after just a few weeks of regular use. Often changes begin almost immediately but it can take a while before you notice. Some people may want to carry on listening to the meditation regularly even when you notice improvements to ensure those improvements are embedded and sustained. It is almost like treating it like a prescription of medication – to listen once per day until you achieve the desired results, for example.

It is important to make sure any audio tracks you make are listened to safely, so not whilst driving, operating machinery, or doing anything else that will require your attention. It is best to listen to audio meditations in a quiet environment where you are unlikely to be disturbed, and where you can relax. Ideally don't lie down in bed when listening to the meditation unless you hope to fall asleep, because sometimes people have fallen asleep when meditating because they are tired. If you fall asleep you are likely to stop being connected to the meditation, and so the effectiveness of the meditation is likely to be reduced. If you can, sit in a comfortable chair to listen to the meditation. It is common for people to think that they have fallen asleep when meditating. This does happen from time to time, but it is rarer than people often realise. One way to know whether you have fallen asleep or not is to think about at what point you wake up. If you think that you have been falling asleep, but you are either opening your eyes just as the meditation is ending, or are at least aware of listening to the end of the meditation but decide not to open your eyes, then you weren't asleep. If you fall asleep you will be likely to wake up hours after listening to the meditation, rather than just as it ends.

When recording or reading these meditations you should read in a calm and relaxed 'non-intrusive' voice. At ',' pause briefly, at '.' pause for a little longer, and at the end of a paragraph pause for longer still. If a much longer pause is likely to be helpful this will be written into the meditation script.

Using these meditations shouldn't be an alternative for proper medical treatment. You should always consult medical practitioners where necessary, and continue with any prescribed medications unless a medical practitioner tells you otherwise.

Spiritual awareness

Sit comfortably and close your eyes, and with your eyes closed take a few moments to begin to focus on your breathing, focusing on breathing in, and breathing out. And as you focus on breathing in, and breathing out notice what the breath feels like as it passes through the nostrils, and notice which nostril the breath is passing through most comfortably. And as you take some time to notice that you can begin to feel more relaxed with each breath, and you can prepare to discover whether you will begin to feel more relaxed with each in-breath, or with each out-breath.

And you can notice the movement of your body with each breath you take, noticing the movement of your body as you breathe in, and as you breathe out, and you can wonder what differences there are in the body as the life giving breath flows in, and out, and as you continue to breathe in and out you may begin to notice heaviness or lightness within your body or perhaps around the eyes, or shoulders.

 And after a while you can begin to discover the breath taking care of itself, your breath taking care of itself as it has for many years, as it knows what it is doing. And as your focus begins to move away from the breath you can begin to get a sense of the world around you, of your connection to the wider world, almost as if you are viewing the world through new eyes. And as you get a sense of this connection with the world around you, you can get a sense of drifting above an African savannah, looking in awe at the vast expanse below you, noticing different plants and animals and the complexity of life around you, feeling a sense of wonder as you discover the beauty of life, as you contemplate that all of this began with nothing.

In the beginning there was no space, no time, no up, nor down, no left or right, no light, no shadows, and now there is life. You can gaze up at the stars knowing you are seeing just a small slice of all that is there, aware that the stars you can see are just a fraction of the stars contained just within our own galaxy, and our galaxy is like a speck of sand in the ocean of the universe. And nature has such beauty and wonder, and you can wonder how you will feel your connection with nature, as you see trees and can marvel at their ability to grow from a tiny seed, into some of the largest living beings on the planet. And we are all born from explosions of stars that happened billions of years ago many light years away, all life and everything you see is made from stardust, we are all one, we are all connected.

And you can find yourself on a purple path heading towards the most beautiful horizon, noticing your connection with others, noticing your connection with nature, with all that is, all that was, and all that is yet to be. Finding your spiritual path of love, kindness and compassion, it can be hard not to be moved, not to feel overwhelmed at times from the wonders around you, and you can notice miracles everywhere, every being alive today is the by-product of a history of miracles spanning back in time to the creation of the universe and time itself.

And you can see the world in a new way; you can see the wonder, the beauty, and the grace of the interconnected nature of the world and reality. We are all small parts of something immeasurably greater than ourselves, yet we are all important, the essence of the whole universe is contained in each and every atom that makes up who we are.

When there is darkness you can be guided by light, guided by an innate knowing, guided by a deep sense of wisdom, by your spiritual awareness. And you can be curious about your spiritual awakening. And you can explore truth, beauty, love and change, and discover a new perspective. And as I quieten down in the background you can take all the time you need to allow this meditation to take place quietly inside.

(You can either have a space of silence for about 5-10 minutes and then finish the session by talking again and saying 'that's it, and you can now take a few moments to drift back out of this meditation and reorient back to the room' or you can end the meditation here allowing the meditator to take as much time as they feel is necessary and they will naturally drift back and open their eyes in their own time)

Chakra realignment

As you listen to me you can relax and close your eyes, and with your eyes closed you can begin to notice the flow of energy around and through your body, and you can begin to breathe calmly and regular as that energy flows and notice what colour that energy has as it flows around you and through your body. And notice how the energy from the Earth flows up into you, while the energy of the sky and the Earth's magnetic energy flows down into you, and you are all encompassed by energy from the environment flowing into you.

And as that energy flows into you it flows in a cycle passing through the chakras, and you can begin to realign and open the chakras one at a time. And you can begin by opening your root chakra at the base of your spine, you can notice a red light emanating from that area, notice how you can feel grounded with the Earth as you focus on the parts of you that are in contact with objects, and how the energy from the

Earth can pass in to you and flow to that chakra. As energy flows to that chakra have a sense of that chakra opening up and notice a symbol of that chakra being open before allowing the flow of energy to move up to the sacral chakra in the abdomen.

Notice as that energy travels up to the sacral chakra the light changes to orange as it flows into that chakra, notice how as that energy flows into the sacral chakra you can become more in touch with feeling and sexuality, and you can take some time to allow that orange light to flow into that chakra before the light begins to flow up to the next chakra, and with each chakra realigned relaxation can increase and you can feel a sense of gradually being cleansed.

And your attention can follow that light, can follow that energy as it moves up to the solar plexus chakra just above your navel and as that light travels to the solar plexus chakra you can notice how the light changes to yellow as it reaches that chakra, and purifies that chakra, and as it does this realignment can help to increase your confidence, your self-esteem and your self-worth, and you can notice the purity of that yellow light.

And once that chakra is realigned you can allow the energy to continue to flow up to the heart chakra just above the heart and in the centre of your chest where the light changes to green, and as the heart chakra realigns you can begin to get a sense of inner peace, of love and compassion, and once that chakra is realigned you can allow the flow of energy to continue to travel up through the body, as you continue to relax.

And that energy can flow up to the throat chakra situated in your throat. And as that energy arrives at the throat chakra you can notice how the colour of the light changes to light blue, and this energy can pass in and around the throat chakra helping to increase communication and self-expression, and as that chakra gets realigned the sense of inner peace can increase.

And you can notice how that light blue energy flows and realigns the throat chakra before moving up towards the head to the third eye chakra at the centre of your forehead, and the energy can change to a pure blue light as it realigns your third eye chakra, and insight, wisdom and intuition can be increased and developed further, and I don't know whether you will notice feelings or sensations as that chakra realigns before the energy moves up to the crown chakra.

And as the energy flows up to the crown chakra you can notice how the light changes to purple and as the purple light reaches the crown chakra at the top of your head it can begin to realign that chakra helping to increase inner and outer beauty and helping to develop your spiritual connection and sense of bliss.

And once that chakra is realigned you can begin to notice how the energy moves and flows and travels from the Earth and sky, into the root chakra, up through the chakras, changing colour as it flows, up to the crown chakra, and then cycles back down through the chakras to the root chakra and back out connecting you with the Earth and sky.

And as that flow continues you can notice a pulsating of energy as each chakra is fully realigned with each other chakra, and that healing radiating light can begin to spread out from the chakras to fill your body, and a brilliant white light can begin to pass up through the top of your head connecting with a spiritual plane, and as that white light passes out of the top of your head the radiating colours of light can begin to flow out from your body connecting you to the world around you, spreading out beyond your physical form.

And long after you finish following this meditation those re-energised chakras can continue that flow in your everyday life, enhancing various areas of your life and touching the lives of others. And as I quieten down in the background now you can take all the time you need to allow this meditation to continue inside.

(You can either have a space of silence for about 5-10 minutes and then finish the session by talking again and saying 'that's it, and you can now take a few moments to drift back out of this meditation and reorient back to the room' or you can end the meditation here allowing the meditator to take as much time as they feel is necessary and they will naturally drift back and open their eyes in their own time)

Enjoy life more

As you close your eyes and listen to me you can begin to focus on your breathing. As you focus on your breathing and begin to centre yourself in the moment you can let thoughts that you have been having just drift by. You can be aware that they are there yet not attach to them, or notice them drift past like sticks on a stream. And as those thoughts drift by you can begin to relax, and I wonder whether you will relax more with your breathing or with the sound of my voice, you can discover that as it develops from within.

And as you relax and listen to my voice guiding you in the background your focus can begin to change, your focus can begin to change from focusing on the day, from focusing on different thoughts and ideas to focusing on how you will begin to enjoy life more. And you may not know at first how that focus has begun to change because it can happen gradually as you relax into the experience further. And there is an old saying 'you get more of what you focus on' and as you listen to my voice and relax a part of you can ponder that thought 'you get more of what you focus on'. And I wonder what you will focus on here and now?

Life is a journey made up of many presents, and each present is a gift to be cherished in the moment. And you can think back to happy memories long forgotten and not even realise you have thought about them, or think about pleasant memories you haven't thought about in ages without being aware of what stimulated those specific thoughts, and we all have songs we can hear that can take us back, and smells that trigger certain happy memories, and places we like to reminisce.

And where you are now is just a stage on your own personal journey through life, your own journey of self-discovery. And you can be curious what it means to enjoy life more, how you will know you are enjoying life more. What you notice when you are enjoying life more, and how you enjoying life more impacts on those around you. And to enjoy life more is to be congruent with yourself and aligned with what is honest and true in the world. To bring happiness to others as you find happiness for yourself. To hold up a mirror and like what you see. To feel a sense of belonging with others, and you can discover how you will feel a sense of belonging with others, how you will develop a deep and meaningful connection with others, and how you will develop from the inside out.

Life develops from love and connection and finding what we need to grow. You can imagine a plant growing, it needs just the right soil containing the right level of nutrients, the soil needs to not be too hard, or too soft, but just right to take hold. The plant requires just the right amount of water, some plants need a lot of water, others need very little to be happy, the plant requires the correct amount of sunlight, too much and it can whither, too little and it won't grow, the plant needs a variety of other plants and animals around it to help it grow. If the plant has all these things it will grow and thrive.

And plants, like all living things, needs to get this balance just right, and each plant is unique and has its own unique balance, and you can wonder what your unique balance is, you can wonder how connected to others you need to be, how you can feel that you belong, what your purpose in life is.

And as you listen to me and allow your mind to focus on what is meaningful and relevant to enjoy life more you can wonder what the meaning of life means to you? What has bought you pleasure and enjoyment in the past, and what you will do to bring pleasure and enjoyment to yourself and others in the future? Sometimes to find yourself is to find yourself through the eyes of others. There was once a wise person that searched for the meaning of life. They searched and searched and couldn't find the meaning of life anywhere. Then on their deathbed surrounded by all their friends and family they could barely speak, so they just listened. And as they listened they heard each person describe how they had touch their lives, their son told them about how grateful they were that they had been helped to go to college, to learn good morals and now have a wife and child, the son's wife spoke about the years of happiness married to the son, and the gift of having a child, and the child spoke about having such wonderful and loving parents because the role model the wise person was for their son. Friends spoke about how they too had their lives touched by the wise person in ways the wise person had never realised.

The wise person began to cry, not tears of sadness but tears of love and happiness. They had spent a lifetime searching, and only now had they discovered how they should have enjoyed life more, only now had they discovered the meaning of life. They felt pleasure and enjoyment from helping others, from being a guide and a role model and they now understood what it meant to have a purpose in life, they understood that it doesn't matter how small their role in life is, bringing pleasure to the lives of those around them and being helpful, that is the meaning of life, that is the path to happiness. They didn't want anyone else to have to wait until they are on their deathbed to learn the same lesson, so they told everyone to go and share my message 'you can enjoy life more by focusing on how you can help others enjoy their lives'.

The wise person's message passed on like a stone landing in a lake, rippling out in all directions touching the lives of many. And what you focus on in life determines the life you get. There are always bumps in the road of life, to challenge us, and your journey is a journey of discovery, only you can discover how you will navigate those bumps and how you will learn and how you will find your way and what you will teach others on route. And the path can be followed by light, and light can illuminate the darkness helping you to discover the way back to the path of light. And wisdom can flow through the path you take and grow with each challenge, with each lesson on your journey as you enjoy life. Without darkness you don't know light, without cold you don't know warmth, without bad you don't know good. Your path is your own to enjoy and one day look back on and discover what made it enjoyable, and I wonder what you will discover and learn? And as I quieten down in the background you can take all the time you need to allow this meditation to continue quietly inside.

(You can either have a space of silence for about 5-10 minutes and then finish the session by talking again and saying 'that's it, and you can now take a few moments to drift back out of this meditation and reorient back to the room' or you can end the meditation here allowing the meditator to take as much time as they feel is necessary and they will naturally drift back and open their eyes in their own time)

Reduce stress

As you listen to me you can close your eyes, and with your eyes closed you can hear what I say and follow along to this meditation, and as you hear what I am saying and follow along to this meditation you can begin to drift inside with the meditation. And as you drift inside you can begin to learn about reducing stress. You can begin to learn about reducing stress by learning how to focus your attention, by learning what to focus your attention on and what not to focus your attention on.

And your attention can currently be on something I can't stress enough, and that is your inner strength, and you may wonder what I mean by inner strength and you can relax, all will become clear in time. And as you listen to me you know I have a voice, and you can hear my voice, and you know you have a voice, and you have more than one voice, like everyone else has more than one voice, you have a voice for the people on the outside, and a voice that talks privately to you on the inside, and you can hear my voice, and when you speak you can hear your voice, and when your inner voice speaks you can hear that speak too. And sometimes that inner voice says things that you would rather it didn't say, and other times it says things you are comfortable with it saying.

And as you listen to my voice you can notice the feelings of your hands and you can have a sense of tensing those hands up a little, and as I continue talking with you, you can keep those hands tense for a while, I will say when to let that tension go, so for now you can pay attention to what I am saying and how I am communicating, because I am teaching you something about managing stress, I am teaching you something about being in stressful situations and being able to be relaxed and calm, and it is all about attention, and focus.

Stressful situations don't need to always bring tension; stressful situations can bring challenges, excitement and a sense of intrigue. They can bring many different feelings, and you can experience stress differently. Having the right amount of stress can help you perform well, can help you learn better, can demonstrate that you care.

And you can let go of that tension now, letting those hands relax as you take the first lesson in learning how to reduce stress. And as those hands relax you can wonder how the relaxation will spread through the body and mind as you focus on change, focus on learning, focus on what to pay attention to and what to let pass you by.

One day in a monastery the head monk went out to take a message to the local town. He told the other monks he would be back in the morning and not to let anyone in. A few hours later there was a loud banging on the heavy wooden door to the monastery. One of the monks opened the door but they saw nothing outside. Unknown to the monks they had let something in. As night fell the monks heard a noise and started to panic, as they panicked they saw a scary shadowy creature in the room with them, when they saw the creature they panicked some more and the creature grew larger. By midnight the creature was as high as the ceiling and the monks were cowering and fearful. In the morning the head monk arrived back at the monastery. He heard screaming and panic, and as he entered he could see the monster as tall as the ceiling. The head monk told the other monks that this is a fear monster; it feeds off of the fear of others. He told them to meditate and to focus on their breathing, to let negative thoughts pass by, to just watch those thoughts and find inner peace and once they have found that calm state of mind to open their eyes whilst holding onto that calm state and keep breathing in that special way as they continue with their day.

To maintain a mindful state where a part of their attention is on maintaining that peace and calm, whilst another part of their attention is on the tasks they have to do and focusing externally from themselves. After a few moments the fear monster began to shrink. It shrank so small it couldn't climb over the footstep at the front door, so the head monk decided to keep the fear monster in the monastery telling the other monks that anytime the fear monster begins to grow they are to calm themselves down mindfully and focus on what they need to do.

As a part of you learns the secret to reducing stress I wonder whether it will happen all at an instinctive level or whether you will have some conscious awareness of what is being learnt. Stress is at the heart of life, it is stress that motivates, it is stress that gets us out of bed in the morning, and stress is what drives us. When we feel hot we are motivated to cool off in a pool of water, after a while that pool of water can feel uncomfortable or cold so we are motivated to get out of the pool and warm up in the sun.

And as you relax and listen to me your inner voice can learn to communicate by focusing on what is relevant, and you can learn that the voice speaks and you don't have to pay attention, you can be aware it is speaking and decide when to listen and when to be focusing elsewhere. Like driving with the radio on in the car, sometimes you can listen to the radio and pay attention to what is being said on the radio, other times you can just be aware the radio is on in the background whilst you focus on the road and on driving, and the radio can be just background noise filling the silence of the drive. And occasionally you can decide to turn the radio off altogether when you need silence to focus or concentrate.

And you can learn from this meditation how to reduce stress and what was meant by inner strength. Sometimes the strongest isn't the fighter; it is the one that doesn't fight despite being provoked to fight. And as I quieten down in the background you can take all the time you need to allow this meditation to continue quietly inside.

(You can either have a space of silence for about 5-10 minutes and then finish the session by talking again and saying 'that's it, and you can now take a few moments to drift back out of this meditation and reorient back to the room' or you can end the meditation here allowing the meditator to take as much time as they feel is necessary and they will naturally drift back and open their eyes in their own time)

Find inner peace

As you sit and listen to me you can begin your journey into inner peace. And as you go on your journey of discovery finding inner peace you can be aware that I am talking in the background. And I don't know whether you will relax deeper to the sound of my voice, or to each breath that you take, or whether you will relax deeper as you become more absorbed in the experience of finding inner peace. And you can listen to me as you relax, and as you listen to me your mind can wander, it can drift to different thoughts and ideas, and you don't have to pay any attention to those thoughts and ideas, they can just drift by, because you can begin to focus on an idea, the idea of walking along a beach with soft white sand.

And you can look out over the clear blue sea trying to find where the sky stops and the ocean starts, and behind you is a lush dense green forest. As you walk along the beach you can notice what the sand feels like beneath your feet, you can walk along wearing shoes, or walk along barefoot and connect with the earth through your feet, noticing the warmth of the sand, the sensations of the sand between your toes. And I wonder what each footstep in the sand sounds like?

And as you gaze over the water you can notice how the light dances and shimmers on the surface and find yourself watching that dancing shimmering light deeply as you sit down on the beach.

And as you sit down on the beach you can begin to gaze up at the sky and wonder what is out there, and as you wonder what is out there, you can begin to discover your mind wandering into space. And as your mind wanders into space you can find yourself becoming more peaceful.

In space there is no up, there is no down, there is no backwards, there is no forwards, there just is. And you can drift in the silence of space with a sense of wonder and curiosity. And as you drift and float and fly through space and time you can explore peace, you can explore tranquillity. And you can explore other worlds.

And as you travel through space as mind leaving that body back on the beach you can find yourself travelling to a new planet, a planet not yet explored. And you can take some time to explore this planet, and wonder about the differences between here, and there. And whilst your mind is off exploring the vastness of space, your body can relax on that beach, with the waves gently lapping on the shore, with the sounds of the leaves rustling in the breeze behind you, and the sounds of birds singing in the trees. And your mind and body can find peace, comfort, harmony and serenity.

And your eyes can be closed as you just listen and relax. And in a moment your mind can find itself floating in front of a painting, before drifting comfortably into that painting to discover a whole new world. And as you enter that painting now, your mind can wander, and explore, and discover, depths of peace previously unknown. And as your mind wanders through the painting it can discover a small secluded hut. And inside this hut is a door, a door to a land called nothingness. And this land can bring peace and quiet to the mind, and you can drift and dream into the hut and find the doorway to nothingness. And when you enter this land of nothingness learning will deepen. You will learn about peace, about how to quieten your mind, and you can revisit this land of nothingness any time you want to find inner peace. And in a moment you can pass through the door and enter that land of peace and tranquillity. And you can be curious about what makes that land of nothingness a land of peace and tranquillity. You can be curious about what you will learn here. And as your mind drifts and dreams in the land of nothingness, so your body can relax fully and completely in your own unique way on that beach, and the body can be aware of the mind yet only as an observer, while the mind can maintain its connection to the body as it experiences peace.

And the mind can learn how to carry that peace into everyday life, how to enter that inner peace while walking around, whilst undertaking tasks, whilst experiencing life. And thoughts can be distant as you experience peace, and you can discover when you can take time for inner peace during the day. And after your mind and inner wisdom has taken time to learn in this land of nothingness it can drift back out of this land and into the hut, before moving back into the picture.

And the mind can travel back through the picture and through space and time to join the body resting there on the beach. And as I quieten down in the background you can take all the time you need to allow this meditation to continue quietly inside.

(You can either have a space of silence for about 5-10 minutes and then finish the session by talking again and saying 'that's it, and you can now take a few moments to drift back out of this meditation and reorient back to the room' or you can end the meditation here allowing the meditator to take as much time as they feel is necessary and they will naturally drift back and open their eyes in their own time)

Be calm and collected

Take a few moments to close your eyes and prepare to relax. And as you listen to me you will begin to learn how to be calm and collected. It is important to be able to be calm and collected when dealing with stressful situations or emotional situations. And as you begin to relax you can begin to learn how to do this. So begin to focus on your breathing, focus on breathing in, and breathing out, and as you comfortably breathe in and out you will begin to drift into a meditative state of mind.

And I don't know whether you will drift deeper into that state of mind with my words, or with your breathing, but I do know that your breathing will begin to teach you about being calm and collected. And as you continue to relax you can imagine walking down a path in a country garden, and as you walk down that path you can notice different plants and flowers, and notice trees and shrubs, and notice the myriad of sounds around you from all the wildlife in the garden, and the variety of colours and shades and textures.

And as you continue to walk down that path I wonder when you will notice the gentle sound of running water from the nearby stream.

And once a part of you notices the stream you can find yourself walking towards that stream, and as you approach closer and closer to the stream, so the running water can sounds louder.

And when you arrive at the stream you can find yourself a place to sit on the grass. I don't know whether you will decide to rest your feet in the stream or not, but you can notice twigs and leaves floating on the surface of the stream, and notice how they drift by effortlessly. And whilst you look down into the stream and become absorbed in the movement of the water and the bubbling sound of the water you can begin to learn about your breathing. And you have a relaxation response, and a stress response, and when you breathe in, this triggers the stress response, it increases your heart rate, it increases blood pressure, it increases feelings of stress, and when you breathe out, this triggers the relaxation response, it slows your heart rate, it decreases blood pressure and increases feelings of relaxation.

In normal everyday life you breathe in and out evenly which means you don't increase stress or relaxation, you remain in balance. When you get stressed you start to breathe shallow and start to make longer in-breaths and shorter out-breaths, this increases the feelings of stress, when you feel relaxed you start to breathe deeply and start to make longer out-breaths and shorter in-breaths, this increases feelings of relaxation.

And you can begin learning here and now by the stream how to focus on your breathing, and keep your focus on the breathing to keep each out-breath slightly longer than each in-breath. And as you begin to practice that, and begin to breathe in comfortably and then breathe out for slightly longer than you breathe in, you can allow your focus to stay on that breathing.

And if your mind wanders from the breathing you can recognise that the mind has wandered and bring your attention back to the breathing. And as you continue to practice that I will continue to talk to you in the background, and you don't need to pay attention to what I say as I will be sharing ideas that will teach and reinforce the learning that you are doing here and now. And as you learn how to breathe in a way that will help you remain calm and collected you can begin to form ideas in the back of the mind about what situations you want to feel calm and collected in, and begin to link your learning about mindful breathing with those situations.

And as you sit and listen to the stream breathing in that mindful way I wonder what else you will learn?

Sitting by a stream breathing mindfully can allow space for peace and calm which can teach other skills about how you think and respond to life events. And whilst you continue to practice that breathing and learning I will quieten down in the background, and as I go quiet in the background so you will become more deeply absorbed in the experience and learn more.

(Be quiet for about 5 minutes)

That's it, and you can take some time to stand up from by that stream and wander back around the garden, and whilst you wander around the garden you can explore different plants and animals with your senses, you can explore how they grow, how they survive and how they thrive, and you can learn about how to be calm and collected. And I wonder which plant or animal will teach you the most about being calm and collected? And you can continue to explore this garden for as long as is helpful as I quieten down in the background and you can take all the time you need to allow this meditation to continue quietly inside.

(You can either have a space of silence for about 5-10 minutes and then finish the session by talking again and saying 'that's it, and you can now take a few moments to drift back out of this meditation and reorient back to the room' or you can end the meditation here allowing the meditator to take as much time as they feel is necessary and they will naturally drift back and open their eyes in their own time)

Deep relaxation

As you listen to me you can allow your eyes to close in preparation for an experience of deep relaxation. So with your eyes closed you can begin to focus on your breathing. You can focus on breathing in and out in a comfortable rhythm, and while you breathe in and out in that comfortable rhythm my voice can begin to guide you on a journey into deep relaxation. And as you breathe in and out you can notice what the air feels like as it passes through your nostrils, and you can hear my voice and can hear other sounds. And you don't have to pay any attention to those other sounds.

And as you listen to my voice you can feel the weight of your arms and legs, and perhaps you hadn't been thinking about them until I drew your attention to it, but now you can notice, when you pay close attention, which arm is the heaviest and which arm is the lightest, and which leg is the heaviest and which leg is the lightest.

And you can learn to pay attention to fine detail, to feelings and sensations that you normally don't pay attention to, and as you continue to drift deeper into this meditation so you can begin to explore how much you can focus your attention. And there is no need to focus on what isn't important, and you can take some time to focus on sensations on your left forearm, really allow yourself to become absorbed in one small area of that arm, notice what it feels like, what sensations you have there, and you can really take your time to allow that to manifest (ensure you give a couple of minutes to allow this to develop).

And now you can allow your attention to settle on a location on your right leg and notice what sensations you have, what feelings you have in that location (ensure you give a couple of minutes to allow this to develop).

And you can explore a depth of relaxation not often explored as you now take a few moments to focus on the top of your head, notice what sensations you have on the top of your head, what temperature the top of your head is, then bring your attention down to your face and ears, notice whether there is any movement in the air touching your face, what angle your head is at and what sensations you have on your face. What sensations do you notice inside your head or at the back of your head, do you notice subtle movements of the head and face, or movements of the eyes under the eyelids?

Now allow your attention to move down to your neck, notice how the muscles are supporting the head, notice which muscles are most tense and which are most relaxed. Notice how that relaxation can spread down into the shoulders, be aware of both shoulders simultaneously, which shoulder seems to be carrying the most weight? Allow the shoulders to relax, I don't know whether they will relax with an in-breath or an out-breath, or relax between breaths.

As the shoulders relax follow that relaxation down into the arms, keep an open mind, allow the open attention to just observe, notice how the relaxation spreads differently down both arms, does it spread with a different speed, or does it spread in a different pattern in both arms, notice how both arms are unique. Continue to allow that awareness to follow the relaxation right down to the finger tips. As the relaxation flows to the finger tips I wonder how it will move into the body. With each breath you take the relaxation can spread in its own unique way.

Once the relaxation has reached the finger tips follow that relaxation into the body, into your chest and back, and down into your abdomen. Notice how the relaxation moves and flows and what happens to the rest of your body and mind as relaxation continues to set in. Continue to keep that open awareness, continue to be an observer on the experience of your body and mind as that relaxation moves down into the legs.

While that relaxation passes down through the legs to your feet you can begin to get a sense of being in a field with a single oak tree in the middle, and as you slowly approach that oak tree you can wonder what you will find. As you reach that oak tree so the relaxation reaches your feet, and with your body relaxed you can be curious how much further your mind can relax. At the oak tree you can walk around it feeling the bark with your fingers noticing the texture, noticing the colour of the bark and the smell of the tree. And I wonder what kind of a day it is in this field?

And as you walk around the oak tree you can notice a small door, with curiosity you can reach for the door, and as you open the small door it can open larger and larger, and I wonder what the sound of that curious door opening is?

And the other side of the door you can see stairs spiralling down deep under the tree. And in a moment you will begin to walk down those stairs with a sense of intrigue and wonder.

And with each step you take you can find yourself becoming deeper and deeper absorbed in deep relaxation, and you can find yourself going one tenth deeper absorbed into relaxation with each count I make from 10 down to 1, and on the count of 1 you will find yourself at the bottom of those stairs at a door.

10, beginning to walk down those stairs becoming deeper and more absorbed in deep relaxation.

9, curious about what will be through the door at the foot of the stairs.

8, being aware of what each step feels like, and I wonder what you can see, hear and feel as you walk deeper and deeper.

7, becoming more relaxed with each step.

6, allowing relaxation to continue to spread comfortably through the mind and body as you listen to me counting down.

5, halfway to the bottom now, yet still unable to clearly see the door down there.

4, perhaps noticing a heaviness in the body as you relax even deeper.

3, almost at the bottom now, I wonder whether you can notice the door down there and what does it look like?

2, stillness can begin to appear through the mind and body.

1, finding yourself facing a door to a land of peace and deep relaxation and I don't know whether you will take one, two or three relaxing breaths before you step through that door and discover deep relaxation on the other side (be silent for a minute or two before continuing).

That's it, and I wonder what you can see? This is your own secret place, a place of deep relaxation, a place where time can stand still.

And as I quieten down in the background you can take all the time you need to allow this meditation to continue quietly inside before exiting this place of deep relaxation and walking back up the stairs out of the oak tree and across the field to reorient back to the room.

(You can either have a space of silence for about 5-10 minutes and then finish the session by talking again and saying 'that's it, and you can now take a few moments to drift back out of this meditation and reorient back to the room' or you can end the meditation here allowing the meditator to take as much time as they feel is necessary and they will naturally drift back and open their eyes in their own time)

Phobia free

As you close your eyes you can begin to relax and focus inwardly on this experience of de-traumatising that phobia. And before we look at the phobia, first you can begin to relax, and to relax you can notice your breathing, you can notice the feelings associated with breathing in, and breathing out, and notice how it feels to have the air pass down into your body, and the difference it feels as it passes back up and out of your body.

And as you focus on your breathing you can let any thoughts that come to mind drift past and keep bringing your attention back to your breathing. And as you continue to practice bringing your attention back to your breathing and letting thoughts pass you are learning one of the skills required to remove the strong negative feelings from the phobia.

And you can take a few more minutes to continue to breathe calmly and slowly in this special way, and any time thoughts or ideas come to mind you can acknowledge them, notice them but not attach to them, you can just let them pass by and bring your attention back to your breathing (stay silent for about 3 minutes).

That's right, and as you continue with that breathing you can imagine a box in your mind, and you can't see inside that box, and inside that box is your phobia, and that phobia is safely inside that box, it is unable to get out of that box and any thoughts that pass through your mind you can acknowledge and then let them pass, like noticing a stick on a stream and then just watching it pass.

And in a moment you will see yourself standing in front of you, and you can watch that you in front of you as they walk around to the other side of the box and as you now see yourself in front of you watching them walk around to the other side of the box you can watch as they safely peer into the box, and you can watch as that you safely and calmly watches the worst that phobia has to offer, and you can watch that you watching calmly and relaxed, and what is in that box stays safely in that box as that you walks away from the box for a moment, and whilst that you is relaxing deeper and deeper and becoming more calm the phobia safely in that box unable to get out is intensifying. It is determined that it will scare that you there.

And you can watch as that you calmly goes over to the box and again peers into the box and relaxes as that you watches the new show, like watching a movie you have been told is scary only to find out you don't actually find it scary. And you can watch as that you again walks away from the box and sits down and relaxes while I continue to talk to you.

And phobias are based on natural survival processes, they are hijacking a natural response, a response designed to ensure your safety. Normally if something happens where you may have been injured your mind makes it so that anything associated with that situation in the future could be a trigger for fear to make sure you panic and run away to safety rather than staying in a situation that could be dangerous. But with a phobia the initial situation usually wasn't dangerous, and if it was dangerous for it to be a phobia it needs to be an irrational reaction to that stimulus now.

So a plane in turbulence can feel dangerous at the time, but a fear of flying because of that experience would be irrational because planes are generally very safe and even if it felt dangerous at the time, or even if you were in a dangerous situation at one time you are unlikely to be in a dangerous similar situation. As anyone with a phobia knows insight, knowledge and rationalising doesn't work to undo the phobia, you need to disconnect the feeling from the stimulus and memories, and as you continue this guided meditation that is happening here.

As the phobia in the box now works itself up to its maximum, and once more you can watch as that you calmly walks over to the box and peaks inside and watches the worst that old phobia has to offer and as that you calmly watches that old phobia you can watch that you watching that old phobia trying to do its worst to scare that you there and notice how calm and relaxed that you is. And that you is using the same breathing technique you learnt, that you is watching that old phobia and any thoughts that might have come up just drift by like twigs on a stream and that you will open the box in a minute, and you can watch on with curiosity wondering what will happen.

And that you there will have everything under control, they are confident and know what they are doing, and you can watch what they do and learn on many levels from what they do. And they reach in to the box and what they find is a book, and the whole history of the phobia is contained within the pages of that book with the start of the book charting the root of the phobia in great detail all the way through every incident that has ever happened to every negative thought that has ever happened right up to the here and now.

And as you watch and continue to breathe calmly keeping your attention on your breath when you notice it wandering you can watch that you calmly flicking quickly through all the pages of that old dusty book from the start to the finish, just looking at the pictures on each page and getting a vague sense of the words on each page and then closing the book.

And then when that you has flicked through to the end of the book you can notice how they decide to get a different perspective on that old book and calmly flick through all the pages again from the final page all the way to the first page of that old book, before then closing the book.

And you can notice that that you is curious and you can watch as that you turns that old book upside down and again calmly flicks through that old book from start to finish with everything upside down before closing the book, and then you can notice how they want to make sure they have checked that old dusty book out from all angles so they decide with that old book upside down that they will calmly flick through all the pages from the end to the beginning as fast as they can, and you can watch as that you calmly flicks as fast as they can through that old upside down book from the end to the start before closing the book.

And then you can watch as that you relaxes in a chair flicking to random pages through that old book, occasionally taking pages out and drawing on some pages and editing other pages, and doing what they can to make that old book more entertaining and pleasurable to read. Some times that you reads a little bit from the beginning before reading some of the end then the middle, other times they read some of the middle before reading the beginning and then the end, and at other times they read the end before reading the beginning and then the middle, and they keep reading random extracts of that old book over and over again until they get confused with how the whole book initially went and they struggle to remember the story as it was once told.

And you can watch as that you goes and puts the book on a bookshelf in a library before walking off calmly and pleased with their work. And as you continue to breathe in that calm way you can go over and find that old book and take it and sit and calmly flick through that old book and take some time to enjoy the changes you made to that old book. And while you do this I will quieten down in the background to allow you time for learning about a new way of responding to situations you once found caused you fear and to think about what will be different in the future without that old phobia.

(You can either have a space of silence for about 5-10 minutes and then finish the session by talking again and saying 'that's it, and you can now take a few moments to drift back out of this meditation and reorient back to the room' or you can end the meditation here allowing the meditator to take as much time as they feel is necessary and they will naturally drift back and open their eyes in their own time)

Speak easy

As you listen to me talking you can close your eyes and begin to relax, and as you begin to relax you can notice that relaxation as it spreads through your body. And as that relaxation spreads through your body you can pay attention to your body and notice which areas are feeling the most relaxed.

And while your body continues to relax, your mind can relax also, and you can begin to learn how to become absorbed in a single moment. And when you are talking in front of others and you want to talk comfortably the trick isn't to relax, it is to be absorbed in the moment, to honestly express yourself and convey feeling, emotion, to have rhythm and colour.

And as you become more absorbed in this guided meditation you can discover yourself walking along a country path towards a gate leading to a meadow. And in that meadow is a calm still lake, a lake that is so calm and still no matter how close you look you can't notice even a single ripple, all you see is a perfect reflection looking back at you.

And as you approach that lake you can notice what the meadow looks like, noticing the grass, the plants, the trees in the distance, noticing the colour of the sky and the stillness of the air. And when you reach the lake you can take a few moments to become absorbed in your surroundings. And you can sit down beside the lake and begin to gaze meaningfully into the water. And as you gaze meaningfully into the water you can notice that you have a curious experience. You can notice that your reflection begins to fade away, almost as if there was a puff of smoke under the water that somehow carries away your reflection.

And as you pay closer attention to notice what will happen next you can see that a new image is beginning to form in the water. And the calmer you become, and the deeper absorbed in this guided meditation you become the clearer that image becomes. And as the image becomes clearer you can notice that it is an image of someone talking to others as you would like to talk to others. And as that image becomes clearer you can notice whether it is someone you know that you know talks and presents themselves the way you would like to talk and present yourself, or if it is someone you don't know, or don't recognise that is presenting themselves and speaking as you would like to speak.

And you can allow that image to form, and you don't have to consciously try to have that form, it may be that consciously you only have a sense of that image, but the instinctive part of you that is learning from this guided meditation will see clearly and learn fully.

And after a few moments you can notice how that image begins to become a movie, and that movie may start by playing something familiar. It could be that you notice the person in that movie giving a talk, or speaking how you want to speak, and you recognise that you have seen that before, perhaps you have seen them live, or perhaps you have seen a video of them before. But after a while you notice the scene begin to change and that person finds themselves in a situation you are likely to find yourself in where you want to speak and present in a specific way, and you can pay close attention to learning without knowing how you are learning, and you can watch them presenting in that situation and you can notice how they present themselves, what they say, how they say what they say, what their body language is, how they use gestures, how they use facial expressions, how they use the pitch and tone of their voice. What their rate of speech is, and how they keep people's attention.

And you can take some time to honestly and fully watch and learn from this over the next few minutes whilst I remain quiet in the background. And whilst I am quiet in the background you can take all the time you need to allow all the learning to become embedded within the instinctive part of your mind.

(Silent for 3 minutes)

And in a moment the movie can fade away into the lake, and almost like smoke changing the scenes underwater you can discover scenes of the future, scenes with a future you in situations where you will be presenting and speaking as you would like to be presenting and speaking. And you can notice in those situations how you present yourself as you speak comfortably, and speak easily. And you can take time to watch that you speak easy.

And those movies that you watch become embedded memories within you, and you will watch movies in that water of memories in the past where you wish you had spoken and presented differently, and this time you will see yourself presenting and speaking just as you wish you had back then, and these memories will become embedded in the instinctive part of your mind, and when you are in future situations where you want to present yourself in this ideal way the instinctive part of your mind will be able to recall that you have a lifetime of memories doing things in this way, and will use this lifetime of learning to help you present and speak in this ideal way in the present situation. And each situation you find yourself in is called the present, and all presents are gifts to be cherished. And some gifts aren't exactly what you want, yet you can still be grateful of the gift and see what you can get from it.

And you can take a few minutes to see yourself in different future situations speaking and presenting how you want to be speaking and presenting, and you can see old memories happen in new ways, and while you review old memories in a new way, and experience future experiences going how you would like them to be going I will quieten down in the background for a few moments. And as I quieten down so you can deepen into this guided meditation.

(Silent for 3 minutes)

That's it, and as you now begin to get a sense of your reflection coming back to that water, you can take a few moments to stand up in that meadow and look around you, and as you do, you can see yourself off in the distance, and that you off in the distance is bright and vivid and full of all of the changes you would like to make to yourself, but because they are off in the distance you may not notice this at first.

And as they come closer to you, they will get brighter and brighter and more vivid, and feel increasingly real. And the closer they get to you the stronger the connection becomes between the two of you. And as that connection becomes stronger so feelings of confidence, fun and enjoyment can begin to cycle through your body, and perhaps those feelings will lead to tingling in the fingers or toes, and those feelings will increase and will cycle back to the beginning creating a loop, and those feelings will spin faster and faster, almost whirring as that you gets closer and closer. And once that you is just in front of you, you can reach out and hug them, and as you do, you will pull them into you, making the two of you one, embedding all the changes here and now.

And after a few moments absorbing the process you have been through you can begin to walk out of the meadow, through that gate. And after you have walked through that gate you can start to feel ready to open your eyes as you find yourself beginning to come back from this guided meditation, aware of how easily you can drift back to that meadow just by closing your eyes and passing through that gate. And when you are ready you can open your eyes.

Beating addiction

You can overcome addiction in your own unique way and in your own time. And as you close your eyes and begin listening along to this meditation you can begin to relax with each breath that you take. And you can discover whether you relax more with each out-breath or each in-breath. and as you listen to this meditation you can learn deeper ways of responding and a part of you can explore what had been keeping that addiction going, it can explore whether it was a pattern of behaviour where the cause was back in the past and no longer applies but had left behind a habit or whether the addiction had been your own form of therapy where it was meeting a need or helping you in some way.

And you know sometimes when a child gets a new toy they stop playing with their old toy and they haven't lost the old toy they still know where it is they just don't want to play with it anymore and I wonder what new healthy toy you will get and all the changes that will happen will be in accord with who you are as a person and will have a positive influence on yourself and those around you and you have experience of not having the old addiction you have the experience of living life differently and I wonder how that old behaviour will become redundant, nobody was born with an addiction.

And as you continue to relax and focus on how you will beat that addiction you can be aware of what in your opinion would be the worst possible outcome of giving in to the addiction, what is the outcome that most drives you to want to change, and you can give that some thought, and ponder that for a while.

And while you take a few moments to ponder that thought you can get a sense of keeping all of your attention on the task at hand. And if your mind wanders you can acknowledge that it has wandered and then bring your attention back to what is important.

And once you have an idea of what the worst negative outcome is you can put that aside for a minute and take some time to think about what the most motivating positives are going to be when you no longer have the addiction, what will be the positive that makes you smile, that fills you with pleasure, what is the life you will have because of no longer having that old addiction.

And you can allow yourself to be absorbed in these positives, allow yourself to be absorbed in this future free from the addiction. And in a moment you will be guided through a process that will change your attachment to the addiction and teach you a thought process to use if you get any feeling of wanting to carry out that old addiction which will help you to be mindful in that moment.

And as you listen to me you can continue to relax, and as you relax you can begin to imagine you are in a field and there is a row of four rooms in the middle of the field, and on the side of the first room is a door into that room, and a short walk straight across that room is a door to the second room, and a short walk straight across from that door is a door to the third room, and straight across from that door is a door to the fourth room, and across the other side of the fourth room is a door leading back outside again.

And in a moment you can open that first door and enter the first room, you will be running through those rooms quickly from door to door and back outside at the end. And inside that first room is the stimulus, or the trigger, whatever it is that leads to you thinking 'I want…' (Name the addiction), behind the second door is a scary room containing the worst case scenario that could happen if you had given in and stayed in that first room, you will want to pass through this room as quickly as you can. The third room is empty, when you are in this room you can assertively shout 'no' in defiance of that old addiction, in defiance against having what you have just seen in the second room. You can assertively shout 'no' as a symbol of the new you that is slamming the door on that old path. And you can even slam the door as you exit the second room and enter the third room, and in the fourth room is the pleasurable experience of the future having quit that old addiction. And after you have been in that room you can run around from the final door back to the first door to go through the rooms again and you can go through the rooms quickly aiming to get through the rooms quicker each time you pass through them.

(Read this getting faster with each round of running through the rooms)

So now you can begin to go through that first door, and once you are in the first room you can run across to the door the other side of the room and into the second room, and in the second room where the worst case scenario resides you can run to the door to the third room and as you slam that door behind you, you can say 'no' assertively and run through the door to the fourth room where you can enjoy a moment of what life will be like without the addiction, and then leave by the door on the other side of that room and quickly run around to the first door again to go through the process again as fast as you can.

Quickly going back through that first door, and once you are in the first room running across to the door the other side of the room and into the second room, and in the second room where the worst case scenario resides you can run to the door to the third room and as you slam that door behind you, you can say 'no' assertively and run through the door to the fourth room where you can enjoy a moment of what life will be like without the addiction, and then leave by the door on the other side of that room and quickly run around to the first door again to go through the process again as fast as you can.

And then again, going back through that first door, and once you are in the first room running across to the door the other side of the room and into the second room, and in the second room where the worst case scenario resides you can run to the door to the third room and as you slam that door behind you, you can say 'no' assertively and run through the door to the fourth room where you can enjoy a moment of what life will be like without the addiction, and then leave by the door on the other side of that room and quickly run around to the first door again to go through the process again as fast as you can.

And then you can follow this process a fourth time, going back through that first door, and once you are in the first room running across to the door the other side of the room and into the second room, and in the second room where the worst case scenario resides you can run to the door to the third room and as you slam that door behind you, you can say 'no' assertively and run through the door to the fourth room where you can enjoy a moment of what life will be like without the addiction, and then leave by the door on the other side of that room and quickly run around to the first door again to go through the process again as fast as you can.

And then a final time during this meditation, going back through that first door, and once you are in the first room running across to the door the other side of the room and into the second room, and in the second room where the worst case scenario resides you can run to the door to the third room and as you slam that door behind you, you can say 'no' assertively and run through the door to the fourth room where you can enjoy a moment of what life will be like without the addiction, and then leave by the door on the other side of that room and then step back away from the rooms and look on a wonder about what you have been learning.

And any time you get a feeling like you want to carry out that old addictive behaviour you can let an image of the worst case scenario come to mind, and follow this by assertively saying 'no' to yourself, and then gaining pleasure from the thoughts of what life you will have because you said 'no'. And you have practiced this process during this meditation, and you can recall and use what you have been learning to make a mindful change to your thinking if at any time thoughts of that old addictive behaviour come to mind. You can acknowledge them without attaching to them, and follow up with allowing your mind to think about the worst case scenario if you had said 'yes' to the thoughts of carrying out that addiction, and you can assertively say 'no' to giving in to that addiction and having that worst case scenario, and then be reminded of the life you are more likely to have having said 'no' and then keep your focus on these thoughts, and looking for what opportunities around you can help you to achieve this life and how much more enriched your life will be making this decision and focusing on these thoughts.

And you can now take some time to absorb all you have been learning before drifting back out of this meditation.

(Allow the meditation to end here and the listener will drift back when they are ready and have absorbed what has been learnt. If you want it to end you can say 'now I'm going to quieten down for a minute or so and in that time you can take all the time you need to absorb all you have been learning here before I guide you back from this meditation'. Then pause for about a minute, and after a minute you can continue 'That's it, and now will all that learning absorbed you can take a few comfortable breaths before opening your eyes and exiting this meditation'.)

Mindful eating

There are times when you appear to be in your own world while you eat and as you close your eyes and listen to me you can discover when to apply the brakes.

And you can begin to focus inwardly, focusing on your breathing, focusing on sensations within your body, and you can learn from this guided meditation about that old eating habit and how you can eat mindfully. And as you listen to me a part of you can begin to explore possibilities and past learning's and even one off events where you instinctively applied the brakes at the correct time without even realising you did it on a conscious level.

And you know there have been times when you have eaten a healthy amount and felt full and times when you have pushed just past that healthy amount and felt bloated, and at these times you have a habit of stopping without even thinking about it, and you can learn during this meditation how to apply this to all of your future eating situations.

And one day you will be in the future looking back at what the main thing was that changed your old eating habits. And you can rehearse in your mind choosing to be very conscious of every aspect of eating, of feeling hungry, of how you truly know you are feeling hungry and not just thirsty or having a feeling that would have led to you eating to fill an emotional hole. Conscious of how you choose to prepare the food to eat, of how you prepare yourself to eat that food, of the process of getting the food to your mouth, of how you put the food in your mouth and how you chew that food, whether you chew the food more with the left side of your mouth or the right side of your mouth, how many chews you do with each side of your mouth, whether you nibble the food and how you move the food around with your tongue, how you salivate as you eat and how the taste and smell manifests into your senses and how much impact each of these senses and the foods texture has on the taste of the food, and what you do with any cutlery or your hands between each mouthful, and whether you engage in conversations whilst eating or focus mainly on the eating, and what speed you eat, and whether you take any sips or mouthfuls of a drink as you eat.

And you can really be mindful of the whole eating process.

And you can rehearse that in your mind, and when you are eating in the future you can be mindful in this way during those times. And you can take some time to see a version of yourself drifting back to a time before any problem with eating began and you may not even consciously realise when this was and a part of you can go through all the relevant memories from that point forwards that led to the old problem eating habit forming and as that part of you works through those old memories it can look for any hidden emotion, you know many people with eating problems discover that when they think back to the events that cause them they remember emotions like guilt and shame or upset and when they focus on those memories a little longer they realise that they also had a feeling of pleasure or control or anger, and the instinctive part of you can become aware of these hidden emotions in the old memories and begin to learn to leave the past in the past whilst learning what is important for your health and wellbeing in the present and future as you form new and exciting habits.

And while the instinctive part of your mind is forming these new habits your conscious mind can be curious what changes it will notice first and consciously you can get a sense of different past situations that stand out and imagine them running backwards and forwards rapidly in your mind with all the action happening rapidly with the speech sounding all sped up and playing backwards and forwards and just notice how the emotion can begin to drain away the faster and faster those old memories flash backwards and forwards to the point where they are just a blur or a flash of light and after a few moments they can begin to settle back down looking similar but seeming so different.

And in a moment I will quieten down in the background shortly while you continue to be mindful of this process of making all the necessary changes to create new coping strategies and opportunities for achievement and learning and practicing to eat mindfully from now on.

And many years ago people used to travel hundreds of miles to scoop stones out of streams and they would work hard to remove as many of those nuggets of Gold as they could and they knew that all they had to do was work hard remove the stones and they would be rewarded handsomely and the job was hard work but they kept the goal in sight they knew that hard work was for their future.

And you know a sculptor can take an ugly piece of rock and they will look at that rock and see the inner beauty and while they hold that inner beauty in mind they will begin chipping away removing all the unwanted stone and as stones fall off the sculpture begins to take shape until after lots of hard work and sweat a beautiful work of art is created.

And you can take some time now to really fully and honestly integrate all that is relevant to making the necessary changes and I will quieten down in the background and you can take all the time you need to allow this meditation to continue quietly inside.

(You can either have a space of silence for about 5-10 minutes and then finish the session by talking again and saying 'that's it, and you can now take a few moments to drift back out of this meditation and reorient back to the room' or you can end the meditation here allowing the meditator to take as much time as they feel is necessary and they will naturally drift back and open their eyes in their own time)

Mindful birth

As you listen to me and close your eyes you can begin to relax and learn about how you can enjoy a mindful birth, and the joy of being mindful during birth. And as you continue to relax during this guided meditation you can begin to explore the potential of your mind and body.

And in many cultures it is the man that goes through the discomfort of labour while the woman just enjoys the sensations of birth and many people wonder how this can be and in many other cultures birth is a comfortable experience the mother only has the expectations of feeling the experience and enjoying the experience yet is not accustomed to feeling any discomfort and I don't know what changes or alterations your mind and body will make to allow you to enjoy the birth.

And many mothers that experience a comfortable birth discover that they were paying all of their attention to the sensations of the experience and the pleasure and excitement they were feeling as they were giving birth.

And as you continue to follow this guided meditation and relax, you can begin to explore how you will experience a comfortable birth. And you can have a sense of sitting under a tree by the side of a gently flowing stream, and you can rest your back against the tree and feel the sensations of the bark against your back, and feel the sensations of the ground beneath you, and you can hear the water flowing and bubbling as it passes by, and as you continue to relax you can learn, and you can breathe in a comfortable way. You can breathe in comfort and breathe out negative thoughts and feelings.

And you know what a warm sun feels like as it shines down on you sat under the tree, and there can be rustling leaves moving in the breeze creating dancing beams of light. And there can be a cool breeze on your skin as you listen to that water bubbling past.

And you can begin to think about when you give birth, you can think about the enjoyment that you will experience, you can wonder about what the sensations will be as the baby moves and prepares to arrive, and what it will be like to experience the sensations whilst at the same time not experiencing pain.

And you can take on a focused meditation state, focusing so closely in on the sensations of movement and breathing being aware this is a new life about to be born into the world, aware of the wonder and excitement at the miracle of life that you are about to experience.

And pain is a subjective experience, people can cut themselves while cooking and not notice until they see some blood and then they feel the pain because they are aware that they should have pain, and they make a decision unconsciously due to the sight of the blood that they should have pain and so it begins to develop. Like a child tripping over and looking over to their parents to know whether they should cry and feel hurt, or whether they should smile, brush themselves off and carry on playing.

And a comfortable mindful birth leads to a calmer pregnancy. And a calmer pregnancy increases the chances of a calmer child, and you have all the skills and abilities within you to have a calm and comfortable pregnancy, to give birth in a calm and focused state of mind.

And people can meditate while walking, while running, while cycling, and doing many other physical activities, and when someone is running and meditating they can keep running longer because they don't feel pain because they aren't focused on pain. They do feel every time their feet hit the ground, and they do feel each breath they take and they can hold a conversation and see the world pass by, but they don't feel any pain, yet if the situation changes and they sustain an injury that needs looking after then they feel pain to make them aware there is a problem that needs to be addressed, and once addressed that pain can go away again.

And a runner was running across a desert and they broke their leg, they felt the pain and were aware of the pain, and then the pain went away so that they could walk to safety, and once they were safe the pain came back so that they remembered to seek medical attention.

And pain is a signal to say something is wrong in this area look after this area and seek medical help. And during child birth there is no need to experience a signal to say something is wrong when everything is going alright. Instead the body and mind can focus on the beauty of the situation. And you can continue to learn how you will have a mindful child birth, and use your skills of guided attachment to decide to focus on certain elements of the experience and in doing so choosing not to focus on other elements of the experience.

You can focus on movements and sensations and warmth and love and breathing and the excited expectation of what your baby will look like, what they will sound like, what they will feel like when you hold them for the first time, and feel their heart beating next to your skin, and feeling their small breath, and looking into their eyes and seeing their first smile, and you don't have to focus on pain.

And your body will be generating feel good hormones and pain control hormones that will help the experience be pleasurable, and help you develop that loving bond with your child when they are born. And each time you listen to this you can learn and practice more and you can take time to sit down, close your eyes and focus on your breathing to develop your ability to focus, to be mindful and to have a comfortable birth.

And you can now take all the time you need to remain in this meditative state allowing what you have been learning to continue to develop for you to have a comfortable birth before drifting back out of this meditative state when it feels right. (Silence from here, most people would drift back after about 5-10 minutes, if you want the listener to drift back quickly you can say 'and you can take a few moments to continue to absorb the learning you have been doing here, and developing your natural ability to have a comfortable birth, and I will quieten down in the background for a minute or so as you do this'. Then quieten down for a minute or so before continuing 'That's it, and you can now take a few comfortable breaths as you reorient back to the room'.)

Increase self-esteem and self-acceptance

Take some time to get comfortable, close your eyes and begin to listen along to me. And as you continue to drift on this journey my voice can continue with you as a comforting part of your experience while you relax deeper into this guided meditation.

And as you follow along with this guided meditation you can continue to enjoy a process of change. And as you continue to relax deeper into this meditation you can begin to wonder how you will develop the ability to improve your self-image and you can begin to make changes on an unconscious level and you don't have to know how these changes will occur.

And you can imagine yourself standing in front of a window, and you can be looking in through that window and see someone that you know loves you, and you might not even recognise that person all you know is that they love you, and you can be curious about how you know that that person loves you, what do they do to demonstrate they love you, how do they behave, what do they think, how do they talk to you.

And as you show curiosity about this you can find yourself beginning to wonder what it would be like to become that person and you can begin to get a feeling of that and as you begin to see the world through that person's eyes you can start to catch a glimpse of yourself and begin to see that you over there through the eyes of this person that loves you seeing what they see that makes them love you so much.

And many people struggle to think of positive things about themselves when asked because all of those positive things are buried in who we are as people and for some people may not be immediately consciously available, and yet these people have friends and family that they know care about them and like them, and these people wouldn't be friends if they didn't like you, and you can think about what they would say they like about you.

Often others see the parts of us we don't pay attention to, and you can think about what others would say they like about you, and while a part of you thinks about what others like about you, you can understand and integrate what I am saying on an instinctive level.

And a sculptor will take a large stone and see the beauty inside that stone that sculptor will keep that beauty in mind and will start chipping away, and they will sweat and work hard and struggle and at times they will want to quit yet they will continue to chip away at it day and night until they have removed all the unwanted stone and they are so proud of what they have achieved and they take that work of art to a gallery to be displayed for everyone to admire the beauty of their work, to admire the beauty of what was buried inside that original slab of stone. And people admire the beauty and all the hard work that went in to creating that work of art.

And you can create your own personal work of art from the inside out in your own unique way, and see beauty in your own work of art created from the inside out.

And looking at a garden you can think that the lawn looks beautiful and that all the grass looks neat and even and all the grass looks the same, yet when you get close to that grass and really pay attention you notice that each blade of grass is different, yet all of the blades together share a similarity and all people on the planet share one similarity and that similarity is that we are all unique and different and beautiful in our own way, and you can begin to absorb the meaning in my words from the inside out as you continue to be absorbed in this guided meditation.

And you can become more absorbed in this guided meditation and develop your focus, you can focus on your strengths and skills, on your positive qualities, on those aspects other like and respect about you. And you can focus on how to believe in yourself. Believe in what you can do and be mindful of what you can't, and you can be confident you will always try your best, you can't be confident you will always succeed. And you have achieved so much and done so much throughout your life, and you probably don't spend much time thinking about it and congratulating yourself about all that you have done and achieved and the positive impact you have had on the lives of others.

And so while you listen to me and at times when you have time to sit and ponder you can take time to think about the good that you have done throughout your life, about the positive impact you have had on others, and you can begin to make this focused meditation on looking back over the good you have done and the positive impact you have had on others and times you are proud of, a regular part of your daily routine.

We often overlook when we have smiled at a stranger and made them smile, when we have said thank you and brightened someone's day, when we have told someone their hair looks nice or praised someone for something they have done. We often overlook times we have purchased something for someone because we know they would like it, not just because we need to buy them a present, or shown that we think of others in other ways.

And you will know what good you have done over your life, what positive influence you have had on the lives of others from the smallest gestures to the largest.

And as you listen to me and develop your self-esteem and self-acceptance I will share a story with you. And each time you listen to this your ability to integrate a mindful approach to any negative thoughts in your head and to any negative comments and actions of others, and a focused approach to the positive thoughts in your head and to your positive actions and to positive comments and actions of others will increase and become easier to instinctively do.

And in a land far away and long ago there was a man that believed he was a failure, he stopped trying new things because he believed he would fail so what was the point in trying. He didn't realise how many opportunities he was missing because he was imprisoning himself by his beliefs of failure. One day he met a farmer that failed to harvest all of his crops in time, so he lost half of his crops and income. The man said to the farmer, "I see you are as much a failure as me?" The farmer replied inquisitively "What do you mean?" "I see you failed to harvest all of your crops, so you are a failure" "I was successful in harvesting half of my crops" The farmer replied "I don't see that as failure?" This attitude confused the man, he felt not succeeding was failure, and failure was a reason to feel bad about himself and his abilities. He asked the farmer "I think you failed, and I think you have failed at lots of things, why do you think not succeeding is success?" The farmer replied "When I try to get all the crops in and manage to get half of them in I know I did my best, I know I couldn't have done better, I am pleased with myself for doing my best and achieving what I did and if I haven't harvested all the crops then I was unable to harvest all the crops, so I am pleased with the amount of crops I have successfully harvested, because I did the best I could. I praise myself on the effort I put in and the amount I have achieved rather than knowing I did my best and beating myself up because it 'wasn't good enough'" The man decided to ponder these comments and think about what a life thinking in this different way must be like. The farmer worked hard, as did the man, the farmer had problems, as did the man, but the farmer seemed more accepting of his situation and what he can and can't change and achieve and this acceptance seemed to help the farmer feel more comfortable within himself, with who he is. The man decided to think about how he could try out being like the farmer for a while and experiencing what a life like the farmers life would be like.

And you can take some time to relax and integrate this learning about guided attachment, about what you focus your attention on and attach to, and what you choose not to focus your attention on and not attach to.

And you can allow some thoughts to drift by, while enjoying being absorbed in other thoughts. And when it feels right and changes have been made you can drift back from this meditation and open your eyes. (Silence from here, most people would drift back after about 5-10 minutes)

Sleep well

Take a few moments to close your eyes, and as you do you can begin to notice different thoughts and ideas that pass through your mind. And some of these thoughts may have relevance, other thoughts may be unnecessary, and sometimes you can notice worries and concerns drift through your mind. And that's alright. And as you continue to listen along to this you can begin to drift into a comfortable meditative state.

And as you drift deeper into a meditative state you may notice that there is a reduction in thoughts and worries that pass through your mind. And you don't have to try to make your mind have less thoughts or worries, this will just happen because you are following along to this meditation.

And as you follow along you can be aware of sounds around you, yet you don't have to focus on these, and you can be aware of feelings within your body and sensations of your body resting there. And this awareness can reduce as you focus deeper into the experience.

And as you become more absorbed in the experience you will begin to learn as a mind and body what is needed for you to fall asleep comfortably and sleep well through the night and wake up feeling refreshed. And this learning happens from within you, so you don't have to be aware of how this happens, or what changes are taking place within you, they will just happen in their own way on an instinctive level. Consciously you can be curious which night will be the first night you sleep the whole night through and you may wonder how you will achieve that. Many people have found that the sleep problems they had were due to worrying too much during the day and going over things in their mind when they should have been falling asleep and they found many ideas worked for them and you can be curious which ideas will work for you.

One idea that works for some people is if they aren't asleep within 20 minutes of going to bed they get up and tidy their home, and within a week they often find the home is tidy and they are sleeping through the night. Another idea is to listen to meditation tracks as you fall asleep to have something to follow that stops your mind wandering and worrying and you may not know what will work for you and you may wonder whether you will sleep through the night tonight or whether you will sleep through the night tomorrow night or whether the first night you sleep through the night will be in a weeks' time or two weeks' time or a months' time or some time sooner.

Many people discover the improved night's sleep develops as any daytime problems or issues become resolved or addressed, and you can resolve any issues or problems in your own way and when your sleep improves you can wonder how life will be different.

And a part of you can take some time to get a sense of what that life is going to be like, who will notice that your sleep has improved, what will they notice, how will it make you feel different what other life changes will occur and how will change be maintained.

And a part of you can drift off into the future looking back and reviewing how you achieved sleeping better each night and looking at those times when you had the odd brief blip and how you overcame those few odd blips and when your head relaxes on the pillow I wonder how quickly you will fall asleep and some people find they fall asleep as their head hits the pillow others find they fall asleep just after their head hits the pillow and some people find they fall asleep after they have taken a few breaths and you can wonder what will work for you.

And as you continue to listen to me you can begin to focus on your body as I guide you through the process that the mind and body goes through as you fall asleep.

So starting with the top of your head, you can notice how the head feels there, and notice the sensations around the eyes and nose and mouth. You can notice the movement of the eyes under the eyelids and the movement of the eyelids, and you can just be aware of the sensations in and around the face as your face begins to relax. And you can follow that relaxation down the sides of the face as the cheeks relax and the muscles around the forehead relax, and the breathing begins to relax, and you can follow that relaxation down into your neck, and notice the feelings of relaxation in your neck and notice whether there is more relaxation in the back of your neck than the front of your neck, or more in the front of your neck than the back of your neck, or whether the relaxation is spreading most down the sides of the neck. And as that relaxation spreads through your neck and into your shoulders you can explore the relaxation as it moves through those shoulders and around the back of your shoulders before that relaxation continues to move into your chest and upper back. And as you notice that relaxation developing in the chest and upper back I wonder whether you can notice the stillness forming through the body as it becomes more comfortable. And you can explore that relaxation as it increases or discover it developing throughout the body as you focus on different areas of your body. And I don't know whether you will notice the relaxation spreads more from the outside of the body towards the inside of the body, or whether that relaxation spreads mainly from the inside of the body towards the outside of the body. And you can allow yourself to notice that as it develops.

And that relaxation can continue to spread down into the stomach area and the lower back. And as it spreads into your stomach and lower back and around your torso that relaxation can begin to calm and heal any anxieties and worries stored within you. And you can take some time to allow that relaxation to absorb into you and through you before it moves into your arms and down into your hands. And I don't know which hand that relaxation will reach first, and you can observe and notice which hand that relaxation reaches first.

And once that relaxation has moved through to the fingertips of both hands you can notice that relaxation moving down into the legs. And as the body becomes totally relaxed, so your mind can begin to relax also. And the mind doesn't have to begin to relax fully until that relaxation has finished filling the body right down to the tips of your toes. And as that relaxation moves down towards the tips of your toes you may notice it spreading faster down one leg than the other. And as that relaxation spreads your breathing will calm and slow down and deepen and your mind will begin to clear.

And as your mind begins to clear you can begin to drift and dream, and as you drift and dream you can discover a pleasant place in your mind, a place of peace and calm and deep relaxation.

And as you begin to notice a pleasant place forming in your mind, like a dream, you can notice what colours you can see, and what shapes and ideas form in your mind. And noticing these colours, shapes and ideas you can wonder what sounds will be there. And as you drift deeper into this pleasant place so you can begin to learn how to drift comfortably asleep. And drifting comfortably asleep your mind and body can be learning what it needs to know to allow you to fall asleep fully and completely at night, and when you fall asleep at night you can wake in the morning feeling rested and refreshed with a clear mind, and I wonder what difference that will make to how your day goes?

(Silent for a few minutes)

And as you learn fully, honestly and completely how to fall asleep at night, how to sleep soundly and comfortably all night long and how to wake in the morning feeling refreshed and relaxed you can drift off asleep once you have made all the necessary changes throughout your mind and body.

(End the track here. If you would like to make this track to listen to during the day rather than as something to fall asleep to then replace the end of the meditation script with 'you can wake from this meditation over the next few minutes' rather than 'you can drift off asleep')

Reduce your anger

Take a few moments to allow your eyes to close and prepare to relax into an open state of mind. And as you relax into that open and receptive state of mind you can begin to notice how focusing on your breathing can begin to open up your mind to change.

And as your mind opens up to change you can listen to me talking in the background. And I will talk in the background about ideas that can be helpful to you to reduce your anger. And the ability to get angry is an important survival instinct. What is needed to be learnt is when the anger is needed and when the anger shouldn't be triggered.

And as you continue to relax in your own unique way I will begin to talk to you and what I say to you, you can integrate on an instinctive level. And you can really begin to explore some issues, and you can do this instinctively, and as you work through those issues I will talk to you.

You know when a car alarm is set too sensitively it goes off all of the time, and a leaf lands on the car and the alarm goes off, or someone walks past the car, and the alarm goes off, and you know if you don't set the alarm the car may be at risk, and the alarm can be set to an appropriate level and it goes off only when it is genuinely at risk.

There is an old tale about a woman that wanted to help her husband to control his anger. She went to the village medicine man and the medicine man told her he knows a way to help but before receiving the answer she must pick three whiskers from a tiger. And on the first day she tried to approach the tiger but the tiger growled and lashed out at her. The second day she sat away from the tiger and didn't approach. On the third day she sat a bit closer and again spent the whole day just remaining still. After a week she had managed to get close enough to hear the tiger breathing. By the end of the ninth day she managed to get close enough to feel the tiger's breath. When it approached the fourteenth day she was able to rest against the tigers belly as he slept. On the fifteenth day she gave the tiger food and did the same on the sixteenth and seventeenth days. By the eighteenth day she had managed to pick one whisker from the tiger, and the tiger flinched. On the nineteenth day she picked the second whisker and on the twentieth day she picked the third whisker.

When she went back to the medicine man and told him what she had done and that she is ready for the answer now the medicine man just told her 'you have found the answer, you no longer need my help'. And the woman went away confused and the next day her husband had changed and was now a much calmer person. And you can learn from this and find your answer.

And as you continue to relax into this meditation you can be mindful of your breathing, allowing your awareness to rest on each in-breath and each out-breath. And as you focus on your breath you can begin to notice how you can control your breathing, and how controlling your breathing influences how you feel. Like the breathing is the link between your mind and body. And as your breathing relaxes and is calm and deep so your mind can relax, and your body can remain calm.

And controlling your breathing can help to control keeping your mind clear and focused; it can help to reduce tipping towards anger or anxiety. And help you to keep calm and focused where previously you may have fallen towards anger or anxiety.

And you can take time each day to practice breathing calmly and deeply, drawing the breath in to fill your lungs completely right down deep towards your stomach, and exhaling the air fully, and allowing your mind to be calm and clear and focused on the breathing.

And you can have a sense of seeing yourself in a time in the past that that you felt anger in, and you can watch that you re-experience that event and notice how things go differently when that you breathes calmly, and remains focused on the breath, and keeps that focus firmly on the breathing while letting emotional thoughts drift by without attaching to them, and if that you happens to attach to any of those thoughts you can watch as that you brings the attention back to the breath and allows that focus and relaxation to continue.

And any time you are in a stressful or challenging situation that would have led to you getting angry in the past you can recognise that, recognise the thoughts that are developing, and then bring your attention back to your breathing, focusing on calmly, comfortably and deeply breathing in, and out. And as you breathe in and out calmly and comfortably and focus on the breathing you will begin to remain calm. And you can practice breathing in a calm and comfortable way every day, and you can listen to this meditation regularly to help the instinctive part of you learn to respond in a new way. And by consciously practicing mindful breathing daily and using this guided meditation daily changes will become easier to discover yourself doing instinctively.

And to learn any new skill takes some time to practice it consciously and with intention until it becomes instinctive. There is a time when babies can't walk. And they struggle, and try to stand, and eventually they learn how they need to place their hands and feet to be stable, before then learning how to transfer that weight to their legs so that they can lift their hands off the ground and start to straighten their back and begin to stand. And initially they are unsteady on their feet and need the support of others, or the support of things to lean on, and after a while they rely less and less on the support and begin to become more confident on their feet.

After months of effort and practice and focus babies manage to walk, and they manage to do this despite the fact that they are growing and changing every day and so they also have to master being able to adapt every day to being a new height with a new centre of gravity, and they master all this from watching others walking, like parents and siblings, and constant practice driven by encouragement and a desire to succeed, and this desire to succeed is hardwired into them, they don't put effort in to try to muster up this desire to succeed, it is just there.

And you can absorb what learning is useful for you and add other learning that seems to spontaneously develop from within you. And as you do you can continue to practice breathing in a mindful way, allowing your attention to be naturally and comfortably drawn to your breathing, like sticks floating past on a stream you can have a sense of letting thoughts drift by.

And you can imagine times and future situations that could happen that in the past would have made you angry, and you can practice in your mind remaining calm, focusing on your breathing, remaining in control of your mind and body and allowing those feelings to pass by and dissipate, and each time you practice this, and each time you do this, it becomes more instinctive, like learning to walk, or learning to talk, or like someone learning to drive or learning a musical instrument. At first it is something you do consciously, and gradually it becomes increasingly unconscious and instinctive.

And you can take all the time you need over the next few minutes to continue to practice keeping your focus on your breathing, and keeping that breathing calm and deep and at a regular controlled rhythm before drifting back out of this meditation.

(Silent for about 3-5 minutes and the listener will usually open their eyes themselves, you can add in a sentence like 'that's it and now you can drift back out of this meditation and open your eyes' after the pause if you want to be sure they open their eyes at that time.)

Reduce anxiety

As you listen to me you can close your eyes and begin to focus inwardly. And as you focus inwardly so you can relax, and as you relax more fully and completely so your breathing can become more comfortable. And you can focus on your breathing, and keep that focus, and as you do from time to time certain thoughts may pass through your mind, and you can notice these and acknowledge these and then let them pass by without attaching to them. And while you continue to relax and drift and become more absorbed in this meditation I will talk to you in the background. And at times you can pay attention to what I am saying, and at other times you can pay attention to what is going on inside yourself, and at times you can let your mind wander and drift and you can just focus on your breathing.

And you know certain thoughts about certain situations can give us feelings of anxiety nervousness or panic, and other thoughts of situations can help us to relax and feel calm. And anxiety is a natural survival response, and in the right place at the right time it can be a useful response.

As you continue to relax a part of you can begin to unpick what situations anxiety is useful for and what situations it is more helpful to respond differently. And you can respond differently.

Many people wonder how you stop panic attacks or anxiety, and to stop them before they occur you can learn to stop worrying and instead start problem solving. And the more you problem solve what you used to worry about the more anxiety stops.

And you can preoccupy your mind and become absorbed in healthy activities and relationships and conversations and as you do changes will occur in your life and people often wonder how you remain calm. And it's useful to remember that a flood of emotion only lasts a few minutes and has to keep being topped up if it is going to stay.

And you can rate this emotion in your mind from 1-10 where ten is the worst and one is the best, and notice how it changes over time and how quickly it subsides. And notice that any response to that emotion also passes. And during negative emotions you can step outside yourself and become an observer while that you calms down.

And you may not know yet how you will integrate this learning, and how you will learn more for yourself. And I will quieten down in the background while you take this time to learn and update the mind and body on an instinctive level.

And you know if a car alarm is set too sensitively it keeps going off and annoying people and irritating the owner. If the alarm isn't set sensitive enough someone may steal the car, and just like Goldilocks discovered it has to be set just right.

(Silent for about 2 minutes)

And some people find that they spend their time focusing on what might happen rather than on what does happen or on 'what if's'. And the interesting thing about the future is that it hasn't happened yet. So unlike the past or the present the future can become whatever you make it. And sometimes this can seem unlikely until you begin to focus on what you want in the future and begin to focus on how you will achieve that, and focus on what you need to do to overcome future challenges.

And over time things improve. And you know at the top of any hill can be a wonderful view followed by a way down the other side. And it's interesting to think that any problem any one person finds difficult to handle there will be someone else that handles that challenge fine. And you can take some time to focus on what you want in the future.

Many people think about a question like that and initially respond by thinking about what they hope it won't be. They think 'I wouldn't have money difficulties' or 'I won't keep getting upset about things'. And this thinking helps to maintain problems. And as they learn this they begin to think about what they actually want and what life will be like as if they are following themselves around with a camcorder. They start saying things like 'I have stepped back and sorted out my finances. I have arranged payment plans. I have sorted out my spending and now spend only what I can afford each month. I have got help that I need. I have looked at what used to upset me and worked out how to handle it. I am planning more. When I notice something that used to make me worry I am looking at what I need to do and planning how I will handle those situations. If I can't change something or have no control over something I work out what I can do so that I can handle it remaining calm. If something difficult happens it doesn't help to also be worrying about it, I now make sure I have a clear head instead. I smile more. I move around more and have increased energy levels. My sleep has improved. People around me seem happier. I feel more relaxed'

And you can think about the changes you will be making to how you think about things, to how you respond to situations, and how you will feel different in situations that used to cause anxiety. And you can be curious how quickly you will begin to notice the changes occurring.

And as a part of you gives some therapeutic thought to what I have said another part of you can begin to learn to relax, and it can take all the life experience you have of relaxing, from falling asleep at night to being absorbed in a good book or film or conversation and can apply this natural learning to the future.

And you can practice breathing mindfully. When you are in situations that could cause anxiety that wouldn't be the appropriate response you can stop that old response in its tracks by breathing in and out deeply and comfortably and keeping attention on the breathing while focusing on responding appropriately.

And breathing calmly and deeply and keeping attention on the breathing helps you to remain calmly in control of yourself in those situations. And you can practice different future situations in your mind while you breathe calmly and deeply. And each time you listen to this that deep and calm breathing can occur more instinctively in future situations where it is needed.

And you can take time to continue to practice breathing in a calm and rhythmic way, keeping your focus on each breath, on the sensations of each breath, and anytime other thoughts or ideas or feelings drift in to your mind you can just acknowledge that you are aware of their presence before letting them go and bringing your attention back to your breathing.

And after taking a few minutes of quiet to do this you can bring yourself back round out of this meditation and gently open your eyes and awaken.

Be more creative

As you take a few moments to close your eyes and listen to this meditation you can begin to prepare to access your deep innate creativity. Creativity is at the heart of being human, and we all have access to this inner resource.

So as you listen to me with your eyes closed you can begin to focus on your breathing, focusing on the in-breaths and the out-breaths, and noticing changes in the body as you take each breath, and as you breathe calmly and rhythmically in that way and notice how the breathing creates changes within your body, so you can allow your mind to wander.

And as your mind wanders you can find yourself on a journey, a journey of inner discovery, of wonder, of creativity. And you can find yourself in a small boat rowing down a vast river, deep in a jungle. And as well as hearing the sound of each stroke of the oar as it pushes water back and propels the small boat forwards, you can also hear the sounds of monkeys calling out in the jungle treetops, and sounds of birds.

And occasionally you hear sounds of movement and splashes in the water, and you know crocodiles hid floating silently through the water, and you know you are safe in your boat. Yet you can still find yourself developing ideas for how you would survive if a crocodile decided to attack. And this desire to plan a creative solution to a potential threat is hardwired and happens automatically.

And there are many ideas you can come up with for how you would handle a crocodile knowing you are in a small boat with an oar, a rucksack, and a few belongings. And knowing you are currently many metres from the shore.

And as you continue your journey deep into the jungle, following the river, you can become curious about the rest of your journey, your journey into the unknown. On this journey you will have to find the location you will be going ashore, and then you will have to find your way through the jungle to the secret temple of inner wisdom, you will have to find out how to access the temple and once inside you will have to find out how to access its secrets.

And this journey will help you to open up your innate creative capabilities. And as you continue down the river you can look out for an area of the shore where two trees make four. And as you row down the river your mind can work on the puzzle and you can notice the sounds around you and the movement of the boat, and the warmth of the sun on your face. And when the time is right the solution can appear in your mind, and you don't have to think about what the solution is, or try to work out the solution because you can be doing that on an instinctive level.

And sometimes the water is calm and sometimes the water is choppier, and there are places along the river where the water is calmer and places where it is choppier. And in some place the air is still perhaps due to a bend in the river, and just around another bend you may discover that the wind picks up again.

And you can be learning all the time about creativity, about looking at situations from a different perspective, about being curious. And you can discover the answer when the time is right. And that answer may remain unconscious the first times you listen to this meditation, and you can wonder when that answer becomes conscious, and when it does you can experience that sudden conscious insight with a sense of wonder.

And when you notice the location you can go ashore, and once ashore you can begin to notice how the sounds change as you now walk deeper into the jungle. And there can be less sounds of the river and more sounds of birds and monkeys, and other animals within the jungle. And you can find a path which will guide you to the temple. And the right path may not be immediately recognisable, but as you look closer you can find the path becomes clearer.

And this path divides at regular intervals, and you can use your innate creativity to find a solution to be able to know where you have come from and you can notice signs that can guide you towards the temple. And as you find your way to the temple, so you can develop an understanding about how to unlock your inner creativity.

And while you walk deeper into the jungle you can find a smooth rectangular black stone that has been gently warmed by the sun. And as you reach down and pick that stone up you can notice what that smooth warm stone feels like in your hand and fingers. What the surface of that stone feels like, what the weight of that stone feels like. And you can notice it getting slightly heavier the more you pay attention, so you can begin to learn how to pay attention without paying attention. And this may sound unusual, yet a deep and instinctive part of you understands what this means and how to do this.

And after a few moments of observing that black, warm, smooth stone while you continue to follow that path your mind can begin to wander, and as your mind wanders you can begin to wonder about how many different uses you can think of for that stone. And you can take time now to allow yourself to become absorbed identifying how many different uses there can be for that stone. And each time you listen to this you can aim to come up with more ideas than the previous time you listened to this. And over the next minute I will quieten down in the background and you can list in your mind as many different ideas as possible and then you will hear me talking in one minute's time.

(Allow one minute silence)

That's it, and each time you listen to this you can find it easier and quicker to come up with more and more ideas. And you can take a few moments to think about how you did this time. And each time you do this you will be improving access to your innate creativity.

And as you continue to listen to me you can continue to walk along that path, and after a short walk you can notice signs that you are closing in on the temple. It may be a glimpse of old pillars wrapped in vines where nature has begun to reclaim an ancient city, or it may be a change in atmosphere as you approach the location of the temple.

And as you approach a clearing you can notice the temple and see a large solid stone slab at the entrance. And you are aware that to move the stone slab you need to find a solution. This slab hasn't moved for a thousand years, no explorer has previously been able to work out how to open the slab, there are signs that previous explorers have tried in vain to break through the slab, and you can take time to step back in your mind and allow the information you are presented with to guide you and to be worked and moulded in your mind until the you find the answer. And you can trust that you will find the answer, and that answer will come from within.

And sometimes the easiest answer is the most creative, and yet it can be deceptively simple. And as you look at that solid stone slab and at the bigger picture, and take in the temple and the surroundings you can figure out how to enter the temple. And you may only figure this out on an instinctive level first, and you may not realise consciously what the answer is until after you have listened to this a number of times.

And in a moment you can apply the solution and find yourself standing in an almost pitch black temple and as you begin to navigate the temple so you can go deeper into this experience of discovery. And what you will discover shortly is the answer to unlocking your innate creativity.

And as you light up the path ahead you can notice how sound travels differently inside the temple compared to outside the temple, there is a silence and a dullness to the sound which is unusual yet calming, and you can explore the darkness until you find the light. And when the light appears it may take a different form each time you listen to this, it could be just a brief flash or a longer lasting light; it could be bright, or only as bright as a candle. And that light can guide you to a book that has remained hidden for a thousand years, a book that holds the answers. And when you find that book you can discover the answer to unlocking your innate creativity.

And you can wonder how you will begin to notice your creativity has been unlocked? You can wonder whether you will get a flood of creativity or whether that creativity will increase gradually, and how much more that creativity will increase each time you listen to this meditation. And you can take a few minutes now to allow the necessary changes to develop before finding your way back out of the temple, back to the boat, and then back out of this meditation.

(If you want to have the listener exit the meditation quicker than just letting them exit the meditation in their own time instead of saying the last paragraph you can say 'and you can leave that book there and begin to find your way out of the temple, and as you do all the necessary changes can begin to happen within you to allow that innate creativity to develop fully. And in a moment once you have left the temple you can follow that path back to the river. And you can notice which route you took to get to the temple, and as you get nearer to the river you can begin to notice the sound of the water and perhaps noticing how the air smells different. And when you get back on the boat you can row away from the shore and begin to drift back out of this meditation and open your eyes.')

Increase concentration

Take a few moments to close your eyes and begin to prepare to go on a journey of inner discovery and wonder. And with your eyes closed you can follow along to this meditation and as you follow along to this meditation you can be aware of different feelings and sensations in your body, and as you notice those different feelings and sensations you can become more absorbed. And the more absorbed you become the more you can find yourself learning how to develop your concentration skills. And the development of your concentration skills will increase as you continue to drift more fully and completely with this guided meditation.

And as you drift deeper into this meditation you can begin to get a sense of walking through a wide open meadow. And in the middle of this meadow is a single grand oak tree. And as you walk through this meadow noticing the smell of the grass, noticing other smells of flowers, noticing birds, hearing birdsong, and other sounds around you. And you can begin to focus on what each step sounds like as you walk through the meadow towards that grand oak tree.

And as you continue to walk towards that grand oak tree you can be curious about what you will discover when you arrive at the tree. And before you get to the tree you can allow yourself to become absorbed in the moment of the experience of walking through the meadow, feeling the warmth of the sun on your face and noticing what you can see, hear and feel. And you can take a moment to look up at the sky and notice whether there are any clouds in the sky, and if there are you can notice what those clouds look like, what size they are, how they are moving across the sky.

And anticipation can increase as you get closer to the tree. You can look at the variety of flowers in the meadow and wonder whether there is more or less variety than you expected or than you would expect in a similar meadow. And in a moment you can reach the oak tree. And when you do the first thing you can do is take a moment to reach out and touch the tree, feel the bark, and notice what that bark feels like under your fingers. And you can run your fingers around the tree and take some time to take in what the tree looks like up close. And you can look up into the canopy of the tree, noticing the movement of the leaves, hearing the rustling they make and seeing the shimmering light of the sun as it shines down through those leaves, noticing the contrasting colours of the shades of greens and browns. And as you look down to the ground you can notices that the area under the tree has less grass and plants due to the light being blocked out by the tree.

And after you have taken some time to explore around the tree you can begin to look for a door. There will be a door that leads into the tree, and the door is a secret door, so you will have to search closely for something that looks different or unusual in some way that gives away the doors location. And after a few moments searching you can discover that door and prepare to open the door and step inside. The other side of the door you will find a grand staircase leading deep down under the tree. And you can look forward to taking that journey deep into the unknown.

And once you step inside that tree you can begin to walk down the staircase. And each step that you take can deepen your experience, and deepen your focus. And you can notice what each step feels like, what each step sounds like. You can notice what is on the walls and be curious about what will be at the bottom of the stairs. The staircase is broad and light and you can comfortably see down to the bottom of the stairs, yet at the same time you can be aware that you know there will be something unusual at the bottom of the staircase.

And as I quieten down in the background for a few moments you can continue down the stairs, and you can be at the bottom of the stairs by the time I next speak, and while I am quiet I don't know whether you will deepen into the experience more with each step you take, or more with each passing second of silence. And when I talk next you can allow yourself to continue to be absorbed in comfort.

(Be silent for about two minutes)

That's it, and now at the bottom of the stairs you can begin to notice that there are many paintings on the walls, and the paintings are all in different styles and all by different artists. And some paintings have special meaning, and other painting can evoke specific emotions, and some can just be intriguing. And you can take some time to explore the paintings, explore the different styles and what the various paintings mean to you. And after some time thinking about the different paintings you can feel yourself drawn to one more than the others. And allow yourself to be drawn into that painting. Let yourself get drawn into the painting, and I don't know whether it will be like you are walking up to the painting and stepping inside the painting, or if it will be like you just float into the painting, or if you get drawn into the painting in some other way. And in this painting you will discover ways to enhance your concentration.

The ways you will discover will allow you to enhance your concentration as you begin to get into a situation you want to concentrate fully in. And in those situations you can find yourself instinctively shutting out distractions and gradually focusing in more and more on what you are doing and you can find it interesting how the more you focus on paying close attention to every little thing you do the more you shut other things out and your concentration enhances, and there is no need to try to enhance your concentration at those times you need it because for concentration to occur fully it just develops by itself.

And whilst that concentration develops by itself you can just focus your attention on finer and finer detail about what you are doing, or allow yourself to be more fully absorbed in what you are doing, and if you are reading you can focus on what that voice in your mind sounds like and how the eyes move and what they feel like as they move and what speed that reading is occurring at, and if you are reading a book what do the pages feel like, what do they feel like and sound like to turn. And you can focus down onto finer detail, and as you do your concentration will increase and you may decide to do that consciously initially, or you may find it instinctively happens unconsciously.

And something in this picture will teach you how in appropriate situations you can prepare in advance to concentrate. You can get the mind-set first and set up the situation and make sure the situation has as few distractions as possible and take a few moments to really focus internally perhaps on breathing or the feel of the air as it flows through the nose and then when you have prepared you can concentrate fully.

And you can take a few moments just to think about those times you have entered that state of concentration even those times it was for just a few seconds and there are thousands of times in your life this has happened automatically without you being aware of it, and you can begin to gather up all of those times and learn from them how the instinctive part of you knows how to concentrate fully. And you can begin to get a sense of how you will know you are concentrating fully in the appropriate situations in the future.

And you can imagine what you would observe if you were a fly on the wall watching yourself in a future situation concentrating, how would you know that, that you is concentrating? What would you see, what behaviours, what body language, what will you hear, how does concentrating in those times in the future make things different, what are the positives of that, how does it impact on your life and the lives of those around you, and you can now take as long as you need over the next couple of minutes to fully and honestly make all the necessary changes on an instinctive level to ensure you can easily and effortlessly concentrate in the necessary future situations.

(Be silent for about two minutes)

And in this picture you can learn how to instinctively focus and concentrate, like waiting with a camera for the perfect photograph of a rare bird. And you may not know consciously how you are learning, because the learning can happen on an instinctive level. And in a few moments you can drift back out of this picture and journey back out of the oak tree and back out into the meadow, and each time you experience this meditation your focus and concentration can increase. And you can practice increasing your focus and concentration every day by taking time each day to sit quietly, close your eyes and focus on your breathing, and practice holding your attention on your breathing for as long as you can, and this will help to increase your concentration skills.

And once you are back in the meadow you can open your eyes when you feel ready and come back out of this meditation.

Relieve chronic pain

Find a comfortable place to sit down, a seat you don't normally sit in that can be the seat for this meditation. And as you close your eyes and begin to relax into this meditation you can focus on your breathing. And as you focus on your breathing you can begin to allow your attention to become more absorbed on the process of breathing in and out. And you can notice how the chest moves, how the stomach moves, how the shoulders move as you breathe in and out. You can notice the sensation of air as it passes in and out of your nostrils, and perhaps you can notice which nostril the air is travelling through most. And as you pay close attention to the airflow in and out of the nostrils you can notice the temperature of the air, and you may notice that the air is warmer on the out-breaths and cooler on the in-breaths. And while you allow yourself to be absorbed into the sensations of breathing you can hear my voice talking in the background. And you can begin to learn how to increase comfort and reduce pain. And as the instinctive part of you learns and develops you can begin to drift off into a pleasant and calming place. It could be a pleasant calming place you know, or a pleasant calming place that is new to you here for this experience.

And so as you listen to the sound of my voice you can begin to learn how you can remove discomfort in the future. And this may sound unusual but you know where the discomfort is, and you know that discomfort is there, and you know which areas of your body don't have discomfort, and you know the discomfort isn't in what you are resting on, it isn't in your bed, the discomfort isn't in any of the seats in your house, or in any seats in any other location. And the discomfort isn't in any room in your house or any rooms in any other buildings, the discomfort isn't in any vehicles or any other specific location, the discomfort is only in that one location you know it to be.

And as you listen to this you will be presented with ideas, and some of these ideas won't match with your situation, and other ideas will fit just right, and some ideas you can adjust on an instinctive level so that they fit just right. And as you listen to this your mind can continue to focus on the sensations of the movement as you breathe and the sensations of the air temperature with each in-breath and each out-breath.

And you know it is a fairly common experience where you put something down for a moment, like keys, and then forget where you put them. And you can search all over the place and discover that you can't find them, yet you know you put them down just moments ago, so they can't have gone far, yet you can't find them. And we all have experiences like this, and these experiences seem to just happen, we don't need to try to make them happen, they just happens automatically.

And many children wonder why adults don't take their hair home from the hairdressers, they would go into the hairdressers and look in a mirror and know what they want removed and the hairdresser would be friendly and talkative and would cut off all the hair the customer doesn't want and then the customer would look in the mirror and be pleased and would then pay the hairdresser and would then leave, leaving an old part of themselves in the hairdressers. And a child asked an adult why they don't want to keep the hair that was removed, and an adult replied once you are pleased with the results you don't want to take what's been removed away with you, you want to leave it behind, and so that's what you do, you have no need for it anymore. The child understood this and knew it was a bit like how an artist may make a sculpture out of wood or stone and they would carve or chip away all that they don't want, and this can never be reattached, and they take the finished item from the work area to put on display, and the old wood or stone that has been removed can never be put back together with the finished sculpture.

And you know that discomfort only exists where you sit right now, it doesn't exist anywhere else. If someone searched anywhere outside of where you are sitting they wouldn't find that discomfort. And you know you can learn on an instinctive level, and you can know how to leave something behind, and you know there is a difference between feeling and doing. You can feel like doing something but not do it, or do something but not feel it. And I don't know whether you will feel like leaving that chair at the end of the session or whether you will actually decide to leave that chair at the end of the session. And I know you are listening to this because you want to leave something behind. And I know that when you leave that chair you will have a feeling you want to leave.

And so many people leave their coat on the chair without realising as they leave a room, and they come back for it, and you can leave something on the chair you decide you can live without. And you can learn more from this on an instinctive level than you ever thought possible on a conscious level, and you can take some time now to integrate and absorb all that is necessary whilst leaving behind all that is unnecessary. And you can learn how you can apply what you have learnt here into everyday life and you know it is OK for parts of you to remain in this meditative state with each breath you take while the rest of you enjoys getting on with life.

And some people find focusing in on the sensations of pain and noticing individual sensations helps to take the focus off the experience of pain. Others find focusing outside of the pain and on something else helps to relieve the pain, and learning to be able to hold that focus where it is helpful is a skill you can develop. And others find what works best for them is to notice the pain and then whilst remaining as still as possible and noticing what size it is, what shape it is, where it is located, what texture it has, what colour it is. And then noticing what happens when you change the size, what happens to the pain when you make it larger, what happens when you make it smaller. What happens when you change the shape, perhaps making it more round, or more jagged, what happens as you try different shapes, what happens when you move it to a new location, even if that location is just a short distance from the original location, what happens when you change the texture of that pain perhaps making it smoother or more rough. What happens when you change the colour, perhaps getting rid of all colour, or maybe making the colour one you would associate with comfort.

And the instinctive part of you can learn from this experience to know which changes to make to the representation of the pain to change the experience. And it can make those changes when it needs to do so.

And the instinctive mind can't be told what to do, sometimes you just need to let it know what you would like it to do, and then let it make the changes itself. And you can take a moment now to ask the instinctive part of you to make those changes and can let it know a realistic time frame you would like those changes to happen within and then let the instinctive part of you do what it needs to do to make those changes for you.

And pain is made up of three components, past remembered pain, current experienced pain, and future anticipated pain. And by being aware you had pain in the past, and aware you are experiencing pain now, and aware you may experience pain in the future, this makes the pain worse. By learning to leave painful memories in the past, and thoughts of future pain in the future you can focus on the present. And as you develop this ability you will be reducing two thirds of the pain even without addressing the current pain. And the more pure you can make your focus on the present the more the experience of pain will reduce. And to reduce that pain further the instinctive part of you can apply what you have been learning, and relaxation also reduces pain, so the more you relax as you do this the more that discomfort will reduce.

And you can take all the time you need before finding your way back from this meditation, and as you do the instinctive part of you can learn how to allow parts of your body to enter meditation independently of the rest of you.

Relieve that migraine

Find somewhere quiet to sit and listen to this short guided meditation to relieve that migraine.

Take a few moments to close your eyes and remain as still as you can. And while you sit there as still as you can begin to notice sensations in your feet, notice how your feet are resting on the floor, notice what weight is on those feet, and gradually allow your focus to go up to your calf muscles, notice whether there is any tension in those muscles, notice what they feel like and whether there is any tightness there. And let all tightness go as you let your focus move up to your knees and muscles in your upper legs. And with all of your focus on those muscles notice whether there is any tension in those muscles and what weight there is in those muscles and as your attention passes up into your lower body you can let all tension go.

And you can focus on your lower body and you can allow a healing light to scan through the abdomen, through your digestive system, allow that healing light to scan into your nerve endings and travel through your nervous system and you can allow that healing light to scan into your blood and enter your circulatory system. And that healing light can get to work traveling through those systems healing anywhere the healing is needed.

And while that light passes through your body your attention can move up to your chest, and can focus on the feelings of your chest moving with each breath that you take, with each beat of your heart, and after a few moments you can allow some attention to move around to your back, to any sensations in your back, like the sensation of the back leaning against something, or the sensation of your clothes touching your back. And your focus can move down your arms to your finger tips and you can notice the weight of the arms, notice which hand is warmest and which is coolest, and perhaps occasional movements and twitches of the fingers.

And after a few moments your attention can move back up your arms to your shoulders and through your neck to your head. And the healing light can continue to travel through all the systems of your body healing areas that need healing.

And while your body continues to relax you can begin to calm that migraine further. And there are often subtle signs that a migraine is due to happen, sometimes these signs occur many hours before the migraine, and the instinctive part of you can learn these signs so that it can put in place a new process that turns those signs into paths heading in a different direction that doesn't cause discomfort.

And you can thank that part of you that causes migraines for being kind enough to give you such a clear message, and in the future that part of you can give a clear message in a more comfortable way.

And as you now take a few moments to focus on the migraine you can do so in a new way. You can firstly take some time to describe to yourself what that migraine looks like, what size it is, what shape it is, what texture it is, what colour it is, whether it is moving, whether it is stationary, what location it is. And you can slowly and carefully describe what that migraine looks like whilst remaining totally stationary, without any movement from your head, from your body, from your hands and from your legs. And you can describe what that migraine looks like in as much detail as possible.

(Silent for a minute or two to allow the description to be done)

And now you know what that migraine looks like you can begin to change it. And anytime you make a change it changes the migraine, and while this is happening the instinctive part of you that knows your entire personal history and everything about you can begin to work on any root cause underlying the migraine to clear that root cause up. And you won't yet know whether that will clear up the migraines for good in the future, or whether it will just make more space between migraines with that space increasing between each migraine, perhaps doubling in time between the migraines, before the migraines just completely disappear, and any migraines that do happen can be shorter each time.

And as you continue to meditate the instinctive part of you can learn to make the changes automatically that you learn here. And one key aspect of migraines is that they are due to an over-sensitivity happening from excessive firing of neural pathways in the brain, and this over-sensitivity and the excessive neural stimulation can lead to discomfort from external stimuli like stress, lights, sounds, colours and patterns and other things, and in some people neural pathways can be stimulated that are associated with specific senses so some people can see or hear or feel things that aren't there, including having sensitivity to touch and needing to reduce the stimulation.

And the instinctive part of you can learn how to reduce the excessive neural activation, meditation can help to reduce this activation by controlling and regulating the flow of impulses across the brain.

And you can take some time to begin rating the experience of the migraine between 0 and 10, with 0 being totally comfortable and ten being the worst it could be.

Once you have this baseline measure start by focusing on the colour of that migraine, notice what colour it is, and notice what happens when you change the colour, firstly changing the colour to a colour you associate with comfort, take a few moments to be aware of what changes with the experience of the migraine, whether that colour makes the migraine worse or better or whether there is no change. Then you can go back to the original colour and then try a different colour, seeing whether this makes it worse or better, or whether the migraine stays the same. You can try a few different types of colour and each time go back to the original colour. Any time a change makes it better the instinctive part of you can remember this and use it to help relieve and prevent migraines.

And you can now notice what the experience of enhancing the colour is, what the experience is when you turn the brightness and intensity of the colour right up, and once you have done this, you can put the colour back to normal, and then reduce the colour right down, fading it right out, and noticing what happens when you do this, before then putting the colour back to normal.

After you have tested the colour you can focus on the texture, focusing on changing the texture to something more rough, and noticing what happens, then putting the texture back normal, and then softening the texture to really smooth, perhaps like silk, and noticing what happens to the experience, then putting the texture back to normal.

Then you can focus on the size of the migraine, enlarging it and noticing what difference this makes, then putting it back to normal, then shrinking it and noticing what happens when you do that, then putting it back to normal. Then you can focus on the movement of that migraine, you can focus on what difference it makes when you increase the movement, making the movement faster, then you can put it back to normal, then decrease the movements making any movements slower and noticing what happens, then putting it back to normal. Then you can increase the size of the movements so that you aren't speeding the movement up or slowing the movement down, you are just making the movement more pronounced, like increasing the size of waves but having them continue to travel at the same speed. And you can notice what difference this makes, and then put it back to normal, then you can decrease the size of the movements right down to any movement stopping, and notice what difference this makes, then you can put it back to normal.

You can next focus on the temperature of the migraine, and you can increase the temperature making the migraine warmer and notice what difference this makes, then put the temperature back to normal, then decrease the temperature and notice what difference this makes, then put it back to normal.

And you can take some time to try out any other changes to that migraine as if it is a physical object and each change you make you can then put it back to normal, and the instinctive part of you can remember what changes reduce the discomfort of the migraine. And you can take all the time you need over the next couple of minutes to do this.

(Silent for two minutes)

That's it, and in a moment the instinctive part of you can make all the changes at once that helped to reduce the discomfort of the migraine and help to make lasting changes. And while it prepares all that is necessary to do that you can just get a sense of having that migraine moving from its current location and floating out in front of you, and as you look at that migraine a couple of metres in front of you, you can begin to observe it, begin to turn it around and look at it from many different angles and notice what it looks like as the instinctive part of you begins to change it.

And as that migraine changes you can notice how all the negative aspects of that migraine begin to form a small ball of light, and that ball of light can shrink smaller and smaller until it is just like a small point of light out in front of you. And as you watch that small point of light you can notice how it starts to get heavier and heavier until it falls to the floor and rolls away from you. And it rolls away too small and heavy to pick up never mind how hard you try.

And after that small ball of light rolls away you can begin to travel in your mind to a pleasant, comforting place, somewhere you can go anytime you need to. And you can take some time to feel the comfort while the instinctive part of you finishes making any changes it still needs to make. And if there are changes you need to make within your life the instinctive part of you can begin to help you identify these so that you can make these changes to help you have lasting changes and you can listen to this as often as you need to fully make all the necessary changes for lasting comfort.

And you can take a few minutes to finish any outstanding work before drifting back comfortably and opening your eyes.

Relieve that toothache

Take a few moments to close your eyes and begin to drift comfortably with this guided meditation. And you don't have to know how to drift comfortably with this guided meditation, or even how to relieve that toothache, because as you listen to this and follow along to what is being said you will naturally become absorbed with increasing comfort in this meditation and will discover how to relieve that toothache.

And it is important that any discomfort, like that of a toothache is properly looked after and checked out by a medical professional like a dentist. Pain is a signal, it is a signal telling you to look after that part of your body, it is a signal telling you to seek help to fix or repair that part of your body, and the toothache is no different. The instinctive part of your mind is there to protect you as a being, it is there to do what is in your best interests, so if you remove the discomfort of that toothache and there is a problem there which should be addressed and is being ignored because you have removed the pain, the instinctive part of you will bring that pain back to remind you to do something about that problem. If the instinctive part of you knows you are getting the problem checked out then you can remove the discomfort and the instinctive part of you will know you are seeking help to address the problem.

If the toothache is a chronic problem and it is just discomfort and not a sign that there is a problem that needs addressing or looking after then you can remove that toothache completely because the instinctive part of you knows that you don't need that signal there anymore.

And as you continue to listen to this and become more absorbed in the experience, you can start to learn instinctively about how to relieve that toothache. And you can begin to focus on your hands. And as you focus on your hands you can pay close attention to which hand feels warmest right now, and it may only be a subtle difference but there will be a difference, and as you pay attention to the hand that is warmest, you can begin to notice that there is variation in that warmth, there is variation in the sensations in that hand, and you can notice where in that hand is warmest and where is coolest in that hand, and as you pay attention to those warmer spots you can notice how they move.

Those warmer spots may move slowly at first, and they may move at a different speed near the surface of your hand compared to deeper in your hand. And you can pay attention to what that movement feels like. And as warmer spots get near to each other I wonder whether they will merge and become larger warm areas, or spread through the hand in some other way. And you can notice what other comfortable sensations you have in that hand.

And as that hand is warmer, the warmer that hand gets the cooler the other hand can get. And sometimes pain can be relieved by warmth, other times pain can be relieved by coolness. And one hand can become warmer, and the other hand can become cooler. And to have relief from discomfort in your mouth comfort can be created elsewhere in your body, before moving that comfort to where it is needed. Like mixing up honey, lemon and warm water in a cup or glass before transferring it to sooth and heal the throat.

And you can be aware of your hands, and notice which hand feels the most comfortable, the warmer hand, or the cooler hand. And as you decide which hand feels most comfortable changes can develop in that hand to increase the comfort. And while comfort increases in that hand your mind can focus on what I am talking about here.

And you know what it would be like to look up and realise that you are in a warm log cabin, with snow and gusts of freezing wind outside, and as you look around the log cabin with the gentle sound of a crackling fire in the background with the flickering orange glow, shadows dancing around the walls and floor and the faint sound of the wind outside the windows you can find your attention drawn to the sound of a whistling kettle in the kitchen.

As you listen to that whistling kettle you can get up from the chair and walk through to the kitchen and take the kettle off the heat pouring yourself a warm drink. And as you take that warm drink back to the other room you can hold it between your hands and notice how that warmth spreads through the palms of your hands, warming the hands with comfort. And that comfort can begin to spread up from the hands to the wrists, and with each breath you take that warmth can spread up the arms past the elbows to the shoulders, and with each breath can continue its journey through your body.

And you can take a sip of that warm drink.

And as you take that sip, you can notice the warmth from that drink pass into your mouth, noticing the warmth from the drink rising up in front of your face as you bring the cup up to your mouth, and notice the warm liquid in your mouth, and then passing down your throat to your stomach. And that warmth can radiate out from your stomach around your body, radiating out comfort.

Once you have taken a sip of the drink and enjoyed the experience of that first sip, you can take a few moments to place that drink down as you walk towards a window in this cabin. And when you reach the window you can look out and see the snowy, blustery weather, and notice the ice on the outside of the window. And your hands are warm and you are curious, you can wonder whether the inside of the window will be cool or warm. You know it is warm in the log cabin, and you know it is cold outside, you know the outside of the window is obviously cold, but is the inside of the window warm like the cabin, or cold like the outside of the window.

And after thinking about it for a few moments, you can reach forward and place the palm of your hand on the glass. And as you do, you can notice what the temperature is and how, more comfort can pass through that hand and flow into your body. And the temperature from that window can help to focus your attention as you notice how that temperature spreads up from that hand into the rest of your body and up to your head.

And that temperature can soothe and comfort that area of the toothache. And it won't take away sensations, only pain, that area won't necessarily go numb, it will just be like a pain dial was turned down. And as that happens you can take a few moments to slowly lift up one or the other hand to that area and this will help that pain dissipate faster and more fully. And I don't know whether it will be the warm hand or the cooler hand that you lift up to soothe that pain as it touches that area on your face.

And you can take your time to slowly move that hand up to the area it is required. And the instinctive part of you can learn how to make toothache fade away by gently touching that area with that hand.

And you can pay attention to how that pain fades, whether it fades like liquid running from that area and draining and flowing away, down to the ground and out of your body, or whether it is like it evaporates away as gas leaving that area, like water evaporating on a warm day, or whether it seems to just dissipate and spread out thinner and thinner until it is too diffuse and spread out to feel it there at all.

And you can pay attention to how that area becomes more comfortable, and the instinctive part of you can learn how to keep these changes going, and how it can make these changes when needed in the future automatically and instinctively.

And you can take a few minutes of silence to let all the changes happen, and that area can relax fully and develop lasting comfort, and after a few minutes when all the changes have taken place you can drift back from this guided meditation and open your eyes.

Boost your natural inner healing

As you close your eyes ready to drift inside and follow this guided meditation, you can be aware that you have a deep inner healing ability. This inner healing ability isn't something that you are able to control consciously; it is something that is controlled by the instinctive part of your mind. And from listening and following along to this guided meditation you can discover that your natural innate inner healing ability is boosted.

And so as you comfortably listen, the instinctive part of your mind can learn how to relax and boost your natural inner healing ability. And as you drift deeper with this meditation you can have a sense of scanning through your body, and as you scan through your body you can notice filling your body with a healing light. And that healing light with fill your body in stages starting with the top of your head. And that healing light can pass down through your body shortly, but first I will share some research information that will help the instinctive part of you to know how to boost your immune system and inner healing. And a series of studies were carried out with school children, they were asked to watch a cartoon. The cartoon contained a cast of characters which represented white blood cells and other elements of the immune response. These children had their immune response measured before watching the cartoon. After they watched the cartoon they were asked to lie down on mats and imagine those characters within their body. After fifteen minutes of imagining those cartoon characters in their body they had their immune response measured again and found that it had increased. In the same way that you can use this meditation and imagination to increase your inner healing response.

And the instinctive part of you can begin to recognise and fight infections and illnesses better, and it can learn from messages coming from the external world and understand that not everything that is different or alien is bad, and some things are actually on your side and there to help you to fight the true invaders and the conscious mind can think about what it wants help to fight and what it wants left alone to do its job and fighting infections efficiently and effectively doesn't mean that the immune system needs to become hyper-sensitive, it can become appropriately sensitive. In the same way that many unnecessary allergies are caused by hyper-sensitivity and the instinctive part of you can understand this.

And as that healing light passes through your body, that instinctive part of you can place a coloured substance or marker on all those bits that need eliminating or healing. And as that instinctive part of you responds in its own unique way you can wonder how quickly positive change will occur, and while change occurs on a deep instinctive level you can follow along to the experience of that healing light passing down through your body.

And you can pay attention to that healing light starting at the top of the head, and as you breathe in that healing light can strengthen. And as you breathe out that healing light can pass down from the top of the head to fill the head with that healing light. And you can notice what that healing light feels like as it passes in and around the head, what colour it is, what intensity it has, and what movement is there as that healing light strengthens with the next in-breath, before spreading with the out-breath down into your neck. And as that light spreads so it can leave any markers on areas to be healed. It can also stimulate your inner healing to improve your ability to respond quicker and more efficiently when that inner healing response is required, like installing CCTV so that you can respond to intruders quicker because you can see them once they enter, rather than having just a few security guards walking around responding if they happen to spot an intruder.

And with the next in-breath that healing light can strengthen. And with the out-breath that healing light can spread down into your shoulders. And as you breathe in, that healing light can strengthen, and as you breathe out, that healing light can spread down your arms to the tips of your fingers. And you can pay attention to the feelings around those hands, is there a tingling, a heaviness, a lightness, notice what sensations are in those hands as you take the next in-breath. And as you take that in-breath, the healing light can strengthen, and with the out-breath, the healing light can spread down through your body to the bottom of your waist. And when the healing light reaches your feet you can have a sense of being on a bench, on a cliff, looking out to sea, breathing in fresh sea air. And with the next in-breath that healing light can strengthen. And with the out-breath that healing light can pass down from your waist to the tips of your toes.

And with that healing light through your body it can scan in the background looking at what healing is needed and boosting its ability to heal in the future. And while the instinctive part of you does that in the background you can find yourself on a bench on a cliff, overlooking an ocean. And as you relax on this cliff you can breathe in the healing sea air and begin to make deep and powerful changes.

And a car alarm is unhelpful if it responds to every little thing as a threat, if a leaf lands on the car and the alarm sounds this is too sensitive. Likewise, if someone smashes the side passenger window and the car alarm doesn't sound, this isn't sensitive enough. You want the car alarm to sound when there is a genuine threat, and ideally you want the car alarm to be intelligent and recognise what is a threat and what isn't. In the same way that you want your immune system to work intelligently and respond to threats to your health, while not trying to attack things that aren't threats. And your immune system can learn to recognise threats, and can learn to take messages from what you consciously learn and know, so if you are told something isn't a threat but your immune system seems to be attacking it as if it is, then your immune system can take this learning and update itself with this knowledge.

And as you enjoy a few moments peace on this bench overlooking the sea your immune system can be strengthened and optimised to respond fully and appropriately, and each breath in that you take can help to keep the immune system healthy. And after a few moments of peace and quiet you can drift comfortably back to the present, allowing those changes to continue on an instinctive level.

Improve your relationship with the one you love

As you listen along to this guided meditation you can close your eyes and begin to drift inside your mind. And as you drift inside your mind you can notice your breathing, noticing how you are breathing in, and breathing out. And as you allow your attention to be absorbed in the way you are breathing in and breathing out, you can be aware of sensations around your face and eyes, and those sensations can spread comfortably down the face to your neck and shoulders. And as you follow those sensations down through the body the breathing will deepen into a comfortable rhythm all by itself, and you don't have to pay attention to that or try to do anything, that deepening will happen automatically, all by itself.

And you can notice the sensations of your shoulders, and allow your awareness to flow down each arm, and you may find it difficult to focus on the sensations in both arms simultaneously, and may find your attention focuses on one arm and then the other. And after a few moments, you can allow your attention to focus on the sensations through the body and then calmly follow those sensations down to the legs and down to the feet.

And as you continue to follow those sensations down to the feet you can begin to form an idea in your mind of the one you love. And this may start with a feeling or sensation or an idea, or you may see them begin to form in your mind's eye, and gradually they will become clearer in your mind. And as they become clearer in your mind, you can begin to notice their eyes and their smile, and as you look at them appearing in your mind's eye, you can begin to get a sense of how the feeling of love develops within your body. And that feeling of love can increase within your body as you look into their eyes, and you can notice where in your body that feeling of love starts and how that feeling of love develops and spreads through your body, and as you pay attention to that feeling of love while you look into your loved one's eyes you can begin to have a sense of what colour that feeling is, and how that feeling moves through your body.

And as that feeling moves through your body, you can notice how it cycles back to where that feeling begins, and once that feeling arrives back where it started it can cycle around again and again, getting stronger and more powerful each time it cycles through your body. And you may notice that there is sound to the movement of that feeling, and different sensations throughout the body.

And as you look into the eyes of the one you love you can be reminded of what you love about them, you can be reminded of happy memories, memories that make you smile. And each time you look into the eyes of the one you love you can experience the feeling of love build and spread through your body.

And you can be reminded of your shared past, shared challenges and how these have helped to strengthen your relationship and connection to each other, and how the one you love has helped you and supported you in the past, how you have been there for them and they have been there for you, and you can have a sense of the shared future you will have together, and all of the good times you have to look forward to.

And you can take a few moments to explore your life with that person you love. You can have a sense of being in the distant future looking back at the life you have shared, and you can take some time to meditate on all those years together and different life events through the ages and how those life events have strengthened your relationship and brought you closer together.

And while you meditate on that, taking as long as you need over the next few minutes, I will quieten down in the background.

(Be quiet for about 3 minutes)

And you can take time each day to notice what you are grateful for being with the one you love, and you can allow that to emotionally touch you, reminding you what you have. And most meditation focuses on non-attachment, and yet there are some things that you want to be attached to and one of those things is the connection you have to the one you love. And you can have a sense of a connection between the two of you, and that connection can be like an ability to deeply and profoundly understand them and feel like you share the same frequencies. And from this deep understanding you can be like Yin and Yang, creating a complimentary connection with each other where you make each other happy and find yourselves attentive to each other's needs and the most gentle touch from them, or from you to them can trigger a feeling of inner calm and wellbeing and feeling of love and strengthen your bond to each other.

And in a few moments you can begin to drift back to the here and now, and as you do you can hold on to the feelings of connection and love you have for the one you love, and you can listen to this as often as you feel is helpful to you. And when you are ready you can find your eyes opening as you reorient to the present.

Open to receive love

As you relax and allow your eyes to close, you can listen to this guided meditation. And this guided meditation can help you to be open to receive love. And you can begin to get a sense of relaxing in a park, listening to the sounds around you, the sounds of distant birds, sound of the wind blowing through distant trees, you can be aware of the movement of clouds overhead, and you can notice what the clouds are like, whether there are just a few wispy clouds, or larger rolling clouds, whether the clouds are high up, or lower down, whether all the clouds are drifting in the same direction, or whether clouds at different heights are moving in different directions.

And you can be aware of the grass beneath your feet, noticing how long the grass is, the different shades of greens and other colours of the grass, the movement of the grass with each gentle gust of wind, the other plants mixed in with the grass and areas the grass is thicker, and areas it is thinner.

And as you continue to relax and drift into this meditation, you can begin to form a connection with the world around you, with the sky, with the ground, with the air, with the sounds, with the colours and the movement, and connecting with all other life, both seen and unseen. And you can be connected with the world around you, and become sensitive to compassion, to respect and to honesty. And this connection can help to direct your behaviour, treating others with compassion, respect and honesty. Being selfless and focusing on helpfulness, always thinking 'how can I be helpful to you?' Rather than focusing on what you can get from others.

And being open to receiving love, is to be open to loving and accepting yourself as a unique individual, and accepting the love of others. And the instinctive part of you can become sensitive to the love signals others give off. And when you receive love from others, you can accept that love.

There is a story about a hungry man, he was living on the streets, he had no money and desperately wanted food. Most passers-by ignored the man, it was almost as if he was invisible, they would walk by and wouldn't acknowledge him at all. Others stopped to talk to him to see if they could help him, but he thought that they were going to judge him, or to belittle him for his situation, so he was hostile to them, and although being a friendly person, he came across as unfriendly to these people, and they walked away without helping him. When they walked away he looked upon these people negatively judging their behaviour of not helping a hungry, homeless man. He couldn't see that they wanted to help, they stopped to talk with him to see how they could help, and they only walked away because of his reaction to them.

To be open to receiving love, is to accept love when it is offered.

And the homeless, hungry man had some people stop and try to give him food, and despite being hungry he refused to accept the food thinking that these people were taking pity on him and he didn't want their pity. He didn't realise all these people were showing love and compassion and wanting to help. Yet he was the one rejecting them. And he didn't realise he was rejecting them, he continued to say nobody helps him, nobody cares, he didn't realise these people were all trying to help him, and were all caring.

And for the homeless hungry man to get help, to get food, he had to learn to alter his perception of reality from one where he interpreted others behaviour negatively and with suspicion, to positively and trusting.

It is easy for people to develop a way to defend themselves against pain and suffering by not letting anyone get close, and this can protect against pain and suffering, but it also protects against receiving love. People can be open to receive love, and this can open you up to experiencing pain and suffering.

But love is more powerful than any pain, love can endure in memories, and across lifetimes, whereas pain fades.

And a mother experiences pain during childbirth, and this is a natural stage to the unconditional love that follows. And many people have many relationships that don't work out because the two of you aren't quite compatible, and the cycle of love and pain of these relationships is part of the path to learning and knowing when you have found the right match. And the pain of losing a loved one is an essential stage in learning your life now doesn't include them, whilst learning that they will always be with you in your memories, and the love between you will continue in these memories.

And these pain experiences are just a stage, they aren't the destination, the pain helps you focus on what is important to address in those moments, once you have moved through those moments, you can be open to receive love again.

And you can take a few moments to fully absorb and understand on an instinctive level how to be open to receive love, and how to recognise the love of others, as well as showing love and compassion to others.

And after a few moments of allowing yourself to be focused on being open to receive love, you can also think about what thoughts and ideas pass through your mind that you can learn to just be mindful of, that you can learn to watch pass by, almost like they are sticks floating past on a stream, or clouds drifting across the sky. And you can become more attached to what is helpful to receiving love, and less attached to negative thoughts and feelings that reduce being open to receive love.

And after a few minutes of making all the necessary changes, you can take all the time you need to gently drift back to the here and now and open your eyes.

(You can also end the experience by saying 'And you can take just a few more moments to make all the necessary changes while I quieten down in the background (then be quiet for a couple of minutes), that's it, and you can now drift back to the room feeling comfortable and refreshed, and open your eyes')

Help relieve irritable bowel syndrome (IBS)

As you listen to this guided meditation you can begin to relax, and you can relax by focusing on your breathing, focusing on how your body moves as you breathe in, and breathe out. Or you can begin to relax by focusing on the sound of my voice, focusing on the pitch, the tempo and the rhythm of my voice. And as your body relaxes, your mind can begin to relax. And while your mind begins to relax, you can drift inwardly to focus on healing and inner wellbeing.

And it may seem a little unusual, but as you continue to relax I would like to talk to that part of you that has been responsible for developing that old IBS response in the past. I would like to thank the part of you that created the IBS response in the past for taking it's time and energy to help to convey an important message to you. And this meditation can help that part of you think of a new more pleasant way of getting that message across. That part of you has all the skills and abilities to develop that new response creatively. And you can wonder what it will be.

And many people remember the frustrating experience of trying to untie knots. And the harder you try to untie the knot the tighter the knot seemed to get. And many people have learnt that, to untie the knot they need to relax and take things slow and easy. And then carefully they can untie that knot.

And the deep instinctive part of you that is always looking out for your wellbeing, always looking out to help you, that part of you can understand, can learn, can develop a new way of managing stress, a new way of reacting to the world around you, can learn how to create wellbeing and comfort where IBS used to be.

And sometimes trees grow large in a garden and need to be removed and you can think long and hard about how to remove that tree or you can worry about what will happen if you don't remove the tree or you can take action, hire someone to help you remove the tree carefully branch by branch until the tree is level with the ground and then carefully dig out the roots one at a time, before planting a wonderful healthy flowerbed. And the instinctive part of you can understand things in a way the conscious mind over looks.

And you can wonder whether you have had IBS for the last time, or whether you may have it once, twice or even four times more, before you never have it again. And you know change can be so quick when change happens instinctively. And you can get splashed by a car and you know to avoid puddles when you see a car coming for ever into the future. And that happens instantly without any thought. And you can learn and heal yourself that quickly here and now and over the next few minutes you can take as long as you need to make all the necessary changes to ensure that old response and old problem remains just as a distant memory. And I don't know whether you will have all the work completed before the end of this guided meditation or just after the end of this guided meditation or tomorrow or next week. All I know is that all the changes will be in place, and the changes will take as long as is right for you. You may listen to this meditation a few more times, or find that once is enough. And only you can discover your own unique route to health and wellbeing, leaving IBS as a distant memory.

And as you take a few moments to absorb what you have been learning, you can begin to imagine yourself walking along a country path, and around you can be fields and trees, and you can notice the grass, and plants, and notice the movement caused by the wind, and while walking along this country path your mind can wander, and you can begin to wonder about the deeper implications of relaxation.

And to remain free from IBS you need to learn how to live harmoniously with the world around you. And living harmoniously is being able to flow with what happens to you. And some people have IBS due to experiencing prolonged high levels of stress, others have IBS due to internalising prolonged stress. In both cases the excessive stress hormones trigger the digestive system to close down because you as a being are perceiving the world as a threat to escape or fight against, or your response may be to freeze and not know what to do or how to react, so you don't do anything. Any time your body thinks there is a threat it stops putting effort and energy into long term survival processes like digestion, and focuses on putting the effort and energy into immediate survival like sending energy to the muscles and increasing awareness. This increase in awareness can increase your experience of light, feelings, movement, and pain.

As you learn to relax and reduce feelings of stress from something that is experienced as a prolonged experience, to something that happens at discrete occasional times where the stress response is needed, you will experience an increase in inner wellbeing, comfort and calm.

And you can increase this wellbeing, comfort and calm by developing your natural ability to focus your attention on positive thoughts, and ideas, on what is going well, and on relaxation and being mindful and just letting negative thoughts and ideas pass by like clouds in the sky. And you can also focus on eating a healthy balanced diet, exercising and leading an active lifestyle.

And the instinctive part of you will know what is relevant from all you have been learning throughout this guided meditation, and what is relevant may be different each time you listen to this. And the instinctive part of you can take what is relevant and integrate it into you as a being, and help you to move towards a future more full of inner wellbeing and comfort.

And in a few moments you can drift back from this guided meditation, feeling a sense of comfort and serenity. And before you drift all the way back to the present you can imagine a healing light passing through your digestive system, almost as if you are breathing in that healing light, and it is passing down through your throat, passing down into your stomach, and down through your intestines, clearing and healing your system, before having anything that needs to be cleared passes out of you. And after that healing light has passed through you, leaving behind only comfort and wellbeing, then you can find yourself drifting back to the room.

Be free from obsessive compulsive disorder (OCD)

As you listen to this guided meditation to help you be free from obsessive compulsive disorder, you can close your eyes. And with your eyes closed, you can imagine sitting with your back resting against a tree. You can be aware of how the canopy of the tree can shelter you from the midday sun. Looking around you, you can notice the grass beneath you, the rustling sound of wind blowing through the leaves of the trees, the stream in front of you, and how the water adds a freshness to the air, and the clear blue sky with just a few wispy clouds passing overhead.

And as you become more absorbed in this experience, you can begin to relax deeper. And you can begin to learn about meditation and how you can apply what you learn to your everyday life.

And to be free from OCD you will learn to change your relationship with certain thoughts and ideas that you have. And as you sit and relax under that tree you can gaze up at the sky, watching those clouds drift by, and as you watch those clouds drift by you can begin to notice how those clouds take the form of certain thoughts and ideas, and some of those thoughts and ideas you can pay attention to, and other thoughts and ideas you can notice drift by as you take in other things around you, like the sound of the wind, or the sound of the water, or the sight of the sun glistening off the surface of the water as it flows.

And as those clouds drift by you can notice that they don't remain stable, they change as they move, one second they take one form, and the next second they can look like something completely different. And you can notice how some clouds are darker than others, some clouds move slow, other clouds move faster, and all the clouds pass by.

And OCD comes from the instinctive part of you trying to do something to protect someone from harm that it thinks will happen if that compulsion isn't carried out. And you can thank that part of you for looking out for you, for keeping people safe from harm, and you can let that part of you know that it doesn't need to do that old compulsive behaviour now, it can still look out for you and be there to protect you, it can just learn that the compulsive behaviour was an over attempt to protect you from harm, like having a car alarm so sensitive it sounds when anyone is near the car, rather than only sounding when someone is trying to break into the car.

And as you continue to follow this guided meditation you can begin to get a sense of noticing a slightly older version of yourself on the other side of the stream. And you know there is a difference between what is appropriate and what is inappropriate and a part of you knows that difference. And as you watch that you on the other side of the stream you can begin to notice as they drift back in their mind to the initial memory that led to that compulsive need. And as you watch that you recall that experience you can watch as they receive all the appropriate and necessary support to heal them of that old OCD. And you can watch as they really recall that experience. And sometimes compulsive behaviours begin with a single event other times they have a number of events and the experience that leads to the compulsive behaviour is an event of thinking in a different way to that final event. Almost like the straw the broke the camel's back. And you can watch that slightly older version of yourself as they explain to a younger version of yourself what the future will hold if they respond in a specific way and what they need to do to prevent that response unfolding. And you can watch as they help that younger you to keep that problem in the past.

And you know sometimes people worry about something happening again and then develop a habit of prevention. And this habit of prevention can be set too sensitive. And while you watch that you being treated you can begin to instinctively process what is an appropriate sensitivity that will let you know any risk is reduced to an acceptable level. And some people get really frustrated with their car alarm because it is so sensitive a leaf landing on the car triggers the alarm. And the owner has to keep going back to the car to reset the alarm. And it can be very frustrating and time consuming. And even when they don't hear the alarm going they are always on edge thinking at any time now the alarm could go again. And they feel so relieved when they have the alarm fixed or set to a lower sensitivity.

And some children learn that plants need water and sunlight to live and grow. And because plants often start growing slowly some children get frustrated and think they must be doing something wrong because their plant hasn't grown into a full flowering plant. And they will give the plant more and more water and the plant can't handle all the water and dies. Other children think the plant needs more sunlight and because the plant hasn't grown enough yet they will give it more light, and then in the strong overwhelming sun the plant withers and dies. Yet the child that let the plant do what the plant has got to do, the child that just relaxes and has patience, that just checks the soil is moist each day and only adds water if the soil seems too dry, and allows the plant light, but not too much light, and if they notice the plant appears to be getting too much light, or not enough light they move the plant to a better location, the child that responds to the plant's needs, these children grow successful plants, and they find it more effortless because they haven't spent all their time worrying.

And you can notice how that future you has been able to help that you from the past, and how they now begin to imagine future situations where that old behaviour would have happened and notice as it doesn't and notice how calm that future you looks as they watch a future you in those different situations. And at times that future you can watch some of the more challenging situations as they rapidly fast forward and rewind those future memories, like fast forwarding and rewinding videos on a TV screen, while they watch until they notice all the old emotion drains out of those situations completely. Then they can watch the situation through at a normal speed in a new way.

And as you continue to relax under the tree and watch that you over there you can begin to imagine what it will be like to be in a variety of future situations that in the past would have led to the old OCD response, and notice what is different when that old response isn't there. And you can notice that you in those old situations responding in a mindful way where any negative thoughts just drift by like clouds in the sky without attaching to them, just being aware that they are there, and letting them pass by.

And you can notice what changes occur because you respond in this new way. And you can notice who else notices that changes have taken place and what others notice that lets them know changes have taken place. And the instinctive part of you can learn how to let thoughts drift by like clouds in the sky, and you can practice and develop your skill at relaxing as you let thoughts drift by, and you can practice imagining situations you would have had the old compulsive behaviour in, and imagine those situations happening without the compulsive behaviour, while you feel calm and relaxed. And the more you practice the more instinctive this new way of responding becomes.

And you can take some time to continue with this experience, and in a few minutes you can follow this meditation back to wakeful awareness

(Silent for 3 minutes)

That's it, and you can now begin to drift back from this experience, becoming more aware of your surroundings, and coming back to the here and now, and opening your eyes.

Improve your learning and memory

Take a few moments to close your eyes and begin to relax, and as you begin to relax, you can find yourself on a footpath leading to the front of a large house with a solid dark wooden door. And this guided meditation can help you to develop your memory and improve your learning. And with each step that you take towards the front of that house you can become more fully absorbed in the experience, and as you become more fully absorbed in the experience you can find yourself learning on a deeper level.

And with each step you take, you can truly and honestly take time to notice your surroundings, you can notice what each footstep feels like, what each footstep sounds like, what other sounds are around you, what the sky looks like, what the plants, grass and trees look like, what the sun and air feels like on your face.

And as you approach the house you can begin to notice the detail around the front of the house, noticing the detail of the masonry, the detail around the windows, and noticing the fine details in the door. And with each step closer to the door you can begin to notice how everything else starts to fade into the background. And as everything starts to fade into the background you can wonder whether the next time you follow this guided meditation the house will look the same or different. And one thing that you will discover is that the inside of the house will look the same even when the outside of the house looks different.

And the inside of this house is like walking into the inside of your mind, and when you enter this house you will notice the layout of this house. You will notice that there is an entrance hall the other side of the door, and many doors to downstairs rooms, and when you walk upstairs you will find many rooms on many different levels, and you may even find a basement.

And you can take a few moments to carefully open that door and walk into the house. And in the house you can find all of the knowledge that you have ever learnt, both consciously and unconsciously. And you can take a moment to walk into a study on the ground floor where you can learn about this house and how it works. Every item in every room has meaning to you, and you may find that you only know that meaning as you look at any given object. And opening a book can reveal knowledge in that book, and references to knowledge in other books. And a lamp can mean more than just being a lamp, the lampshade may mean one thing, while the light may mean something else.

And some things will have special meaning because they represent or symbolise knowledge, other things will have clearer meaning. And all of it is created by the deep instinctive part of you, the part of you that learns and contains all of your knowledge and wisdom. And sometimes something will be remembered because of a journey around a room or a journey around a series of objects in a room, or even on a table. It could be looking at a coffee table and seeing a cup, a large hardback book, a notepad with some doodles drawn on it, a vase with flowers in it, and a few other objects. And each object can have significance for remembering as individual objects, and the objects together can help recall other information. And you can use this house like a memory palace to store and recall information, knowing anytime you want to recall something you can visit the relevant room and look through the objects and find the information. And with practice the process of storing and recalling information can get easier.

And you can have an instinctive knowledge of the layout of this house, and like all properties you can find new stuff and acquire new stuff, it can be new books, new ornaments, and many other new items, and each time you get new items you can find a home in this house for those items. And the layout of each room will make sense to you, and you can take as long as you like to explore the layout of this house.

And as you explore each floor, and each room perhaps you will find that there is a room dedicated to different things, like a room dedicated to numbers, a room dedicated to names, a room dedicated to specific subjects, and you can visit this house anytime you like by just closing your eyes and walking up to the front door, and opening the door.

And when you are learning information you can be aware of the state of mind you are in at the time you are learning or absorbing information that you hope to learn, and you can think of specific pieces of music, or listen to specific pieces of music as you learn something so that to recall that information you can recall the music and that state of mind, so for example if you were learning for an exam, you can learn whilst feeling calm and relaxed and listening to a specific piece of classical music, and then in the exam you can put yourself into that relaxed state and recall that same piece of music and you will be opening the doors to accessing the information you learnt, and you will then be able to recall it. And with practice you will find this easier and easier to do.

And memory is state-dependant, which means that the state of mind you are in when you learn something is the state of mind that is encoded with the memory, so the easiest way to recall that information is to be back in that state. And the more senses involved in creating that state the easier it is to recall, so having a sound, having sights, having a smell, and a feeling makes memory recall easiest.

And so if you learn something when you are relaxed, you need to be relaxed at the time you need to recall it, and you can focus on relaxing your breathing or focus on mindful awareness and not attaching to negative or worrying thoughts. One of the main reasons for failing to recall the required information during an exam is because the person is stressed in the exam, yet they were calm at home when they were learning. So to overcome this and recall the required information they need to relax.

And with a memory mansion, and by actively focusing on how you encode memories in your brain when you learn, you can increase your ability to learn, and your ability to recall information. And as you listen to this meditation and continue to just explore that house you can begin to develop a shorthand, like using keywords that remind you of larger chunks of information. And this can develop each time you listen to this meditation, and the more you practice this and use these techniques.

And you will also improve your ability to control your focus of attention, from learning something, to briefly going inside your mind to place that new knowledge into the relevant location in your memory mansion, to focusing back out on what you are learning next. And then when you recall information you can focus externally on identifying what you need to recall, and then focus internally briefly on where that information will be stored, before focusing externally again with the required information.

And with regular practice and regular use of this guided meditation, and regular trips into your memory mansion, you can improve and develop this skill and it will begin to become automatic.

And for now you can take some time to explore your memory mansion, deciding where things will go, and you may discover new rooms at times when you revisit the mansion where new categories of information are stored, and for now you can take some time to decide on the initial rooms and how they should be decorated and where things should go, and each time you listen to this or visit your memory mansion you can build on previous work you have done. And you can take as long as you like over the next five minutes to do that.

(Silent for 5 minutes)

And now you can find your way back out of the mansion and back out onto that path, and once you are back out onto the path, you can take a few moments to walk back up the path as you drift back to wakeful awareness and open your eyes.

Find a path in life & attract success

Take a few moments to close your eyes as you listen to this guided meditation. And with your eyes closed have a sense that you are surrounded by a universal energy, and to begin with you can go through a process of drawing in some of that universal energy. So pay attention to the top of your head, get a feeling for what you can notice about the top of your head, perhaps the feeling of the air around your head, or perhaps hair on your head, or other sensations, and begin to notice light around the top of your head, and notice how the light is coloured, notice how the light is shimmering, and have a sense of recognising that that light is the light of the universe, it is the light from all of the energy of the universe, and as it passes down through you, it will begin to make you a part of the universe as well, it will begin to synchronise you with the rest of the universe.

And have a sense of that light relaxing its way down from the top of your head, down through your face, through your cheeks, around the eyes, softening as it goes, relaxing those muscles. And allow yourself to follow that light as it spreads down towards your neck as it softens out over your shoulders and down your arms, and you can be curious which arm it is going to soften into first, which arm the light will move into the fastest.

And you can notice whether it moves fastest down the right side or the left side. And you can notice how the light can soften its way down your body, perhaps faster down the front of your body than the back of your body, or perhaps you will notice it soften its way down the back faster than the front of your body, as that light softens through your body comfortably. And that light can comfortably pass through the chest, and comfortably begin to fill your organs with that universal energy.

And as that light flows down towards your stomach you may begin to notice how the light has a sensation to it as it comfortably continues to spread down to your hips, to the tops of your legs. And a part of you can be curious to discover where you are going to end up inside your mind in a little while as that light continues to spread down your legs all the way down to your feet, so comfortably all the way down to your feet. And as you take a few moments to really get a sense of how that fills up joining you with the rest of the universe.

And perhaps there can be some tingling or a heaviness or a numbness within your body as that energy continues to flow. And as that light continues to maintain a level of comfort and continues to move around your body, relaxing your body and mind a part of you that is attached to that universal energy, to the universal consciousness can begin to create a path in your mind. And in a moment you can walk down that path, and at the end of that path is a door way, an entrance, and inscribed on that entrance is a multitude of symbols and words, like comfort, excitement, enlightenment, reality, discovery, wonder.

And you can wonder what else will be on that door when you have wandered down to that entrance and you can be curious about what will be on the other side, and you can now begin to take the steps towards that entrance. And you can get a sense of what is around the path, whether the path is along a beach, through woodland or a forest, through mountains, or through a country garden, and you can look around and see where the path is.

And as you walk towards that door you can begin to discover how many steps it will take to get there, it could be ten steps, or twenty steps or thirty steps or some other amount of steps, and with each step you take a part of you can go deeper and deeper into this experience, into that state of mind that is necessary to plan your future.

And with each step you take you can go deeper and deeper into that state that is ideal for creating and planning future events. And you can now take some time to walk towards that entrance, and when that time passes you can discover yourself at that entrance looking forward to getting through the entrance, curious about what is the other side.

And when you reach the entrance it will feel so natural and relaxing and you can wait at the entrance until the time is right for you to enter.

(Silent for 2 minutes)

As you now prepare yourself for passing through that entrance, and in your own time you can step through the entrance and meet a genii there, and you can be curious what the genii will look like. The genii can take many forms. For some people the genii looks like an animal, others discover the genii is more like a presence in the room, or in that place. And the genii can grant an unlimited number of wishes.

So now you can take as long as you need over the next five minutes to have a sense of the future that you would like to happen as if you are looking back over many years of your life. And you can look back over key events from all of that time, or look over key events from each year, or it could be significant stages over the years, or just a few of the memories that stand out. And you can explore what your path in life is, who do you want to become, how do you want to be remembered, what do you want to be remembered for, what do you want your legacy to be, and how will you make this legacy happen.

You can explore what the first steps are towards that future legacy, and what you will be doing in six months' time, in a years' time, in three years' time, in five years' time, and other times off into the future. And when you are off in the future looking back on your life you can think about what you were doing to have a sense of purpose, to have a feeling of belonging, to feel a sense of achievement and direction with your life, to feel a connection with others.

And as you do that, you can make sure to fully and honestly believe that those events are true, that they are happening as you are thinking about them and that they can happen, and you can go through those events as if they are happening right now, seeing what you will see, hearing what you will hear, and feeling what you will feel, so that on an instinctive level you will seek out in the future to match the patterns of those events, to help those events become a self-fulfilling prophecy.

If you say to someone 'don't think of a pink elephant' you have created a pattern of something to look out for, so they keep thinking of a pink elephant. If you tell someone 'don't drop those glasses' this creates a pattern for the instinctive part of them to follow, and increases the chances of them dropping the glasses. If you tell someone to imagine playing golf like Tiger Woods, this lays down the pattern for them to play better golf in the future. And you want to meditate on what is useful for your future, what patterns you would like to drive your future actions, and what patterns will be active increasing your focus of attention on noticing anything in the direction of those patterns.

If someone believes they are unlucky they will walk past money on the ground and not notice it because the pattern they are working from is to not see the money so that they can remain unlucky. If they believe they are lucky they will see the money and pick it up. Both people have the same opportunities, but only the person with the patterns activated to notice opportunities notices the money.

(Silent for 5 minutes)

That's it, and you can listen to this as often as you like to come back to this place to work on laying down the patterns for anything you want in the future that is within your control. Helping you to be successful, to be wealthy, to be happy and healthy.

And you can now take time to leave through that door again and walk back along the path towards wakeful awareness. And as you leave this place and walk back along that path the instinctive part of you can integrate everything you have been doing, making all the necessary changes to ensure those patterns are in place, and a part of you can remain focused on following your path to the success you want in the future. And as you walk back along that path the light can leave your body from your feet up as you drift back to the here and now and open your eyes.

Forgiveness

Take a few moments to close your eyes, and begin to focus on your breathing a moment, focus on breathing in, and breathing out, and you can be aware of sounds around you, you can be aware of what it feels like to be relaxing there, and every now and then certain thoughts and images can come to mind, and some of them will just drift away again as you listen to this.

And you can get a sense of walking down a path, walking down a path through a nice countryside area, and you can be aware of the sounds of birds, you can be aware of the feeling of the breeze on your face and the warmth of the sun on your skin. And as you walk down this path you can be aware of country smells and the blue sky, perhaps you can notice a few white wispy clouds.

And as you drift into this journey, you can comfortably follow this guided meditation. And you can continue to enjoy this process of change. And you can be aware of a bench off in the distance. And you can walk towards that bench, and you can sit down comfortably on that bench as you drift deeper into this experience. And you can look around and notice the view from the bench, noticing what you can see, what you can hear, noticing what it feels like to be sat on that bench there.

And you can have a sense of drifting up out of your body sat there on that bench, drifting up out of your body, and off to the side over behind some nearby bushes looking over at that you sat on that bench. And you can notice how much more absorbing the experience can be from this perspective being curious, wondering what will happen next, wondering who is going to come and sit next to you on that bench over there.

You don't have to know exactly who that somebody is, but somebody wanting forgiveness, somebody who is wanting to be forgiven. And you can just get a sense of watching that you over there on that bench doing what they have to do to forgive that person who sits down with them. And you don't have to just be aware of that you sat over there with that person they are about to forgive. You can also be aware of something odd that happens, a light seems to come up off of the shoulders up into the sky. The light just seems to lift as that forgiveness is given.

And you know as the story goes that one of the criminals on the cross next to Jesus asked for forgiveness and Jesus gave that forgiveness and that man got the chance to go to heaven. And you know in all religions forgiveness is a huge part of those religions. To have the strength to be able to forgive somebody for whatever they have done.

And just get a sense of watching that you over there forgiving that person that has sat down with them. And you can watch what happens as that you forgive that person. Watch the positive outcome of it., watch how you know the moment they are forgiven and then just get a sense of how you know that that you there has forgiven that person, notice how you know they are now happier as a person.

And you can get a sense, almost like you have x-ray vision and you can see into them. And you can see that the way your genes are expressed are changing to calm relaxed settings, that not only has that you done something good for yourself but also done something good for future generations, and for those people that that you interacts with.

And then as the you over here watching that you over there, get a sense of thinking wouldn't it be nice to know what it felt like for that you over there to do what they just did. And as you think that to yourself get a sense of drifting into that you over there before that other person had come out and joined them. Perhaps there is butterflies in the stomach from anticipation because you know someone is about to come out and join you and you know you are about to forgive them. And you are nervous about what it is going to feel like, how that pleasant feeling is going to happen when you forgive that person, what it is going to feel like to have that light lifting off your shoulders, what all the physical changes throughout your body will feel like, and changes in the mind.

And get a sense of that person coming out and sitting next to you and asking to be forgiven. And get a sense of forgiving that person and letting go. Yet remembering you are not forgetting what they did. You are allowing them to own their own problem and live with what they did. And you can know that within yourself you are making the right decision leaving them with their guilt, and leaving them holding full responsibility for their own actions.

And after that light has lifted off your shoulders and that person has got up and walked off you can have a sense of leaving the bench and all that behind you as you drift deeper into your mind to learn from this experience before you will drift back out of this guided meditation and back to the here and now.

Loving kindness meditation

As you listen to this you can close your eyes and begin to drift inside, and as you begin to drift inside with your eyes closed, you can begin to become absorbed in the sounds around you, absorbed in thoughts and associations that come to mind. And you can focus on this experience more fully as you become more fully absorbed. And you can begin to focus on the point just behind your nose where you can notice the warmth or coolness of each in-breath and each out-breath. And you can focus on each in-breath and each out-breath, and as you continue to pay attention to each in-breath and each out-breath you can begin to notice the sensation of a specific colour that can begin to flow in with each in-breath, while any negativity can begin to flow out with each out-breath. And you can discover how that colour begins to fill your body, it may fill your body from the feet upwards, or from the head downwards, or from the heart outwards, or perhaps it will spread from the lungs.

And that colour won't just fill up being confined to your physical body, it will spread to your spiritual self as well. It will truly and honestly begin to spread and radiate from you.

And the more you continue to breathe in that way, the more the loving kindness, that light, that colour can radiate from your heart, and it may feel like it is radiating from elsewhere, and as that loving kindness radiates from your heart, that sense of loving kindness can begin to grow. And you know what it is like when you are out walking perhaps through the countryside, or elsewhere and you see a sick animal, and you just feel an overwhelming urge to go over to help it with that strong desire to want to heal that animal.

And in your mind you can begin to experience what it is like to have a healing presence, to have healing hands, to have a healing touch, that seems totally instinctive, that seems to be a part of you. And with each breath as that becomes more a part of you, any negativity can begin to become apart from you. And the more negativity you breathe out the more loving kindness you can breathe in. And the more you breathe in this special way, especially when you are feeling drained and tired the more recharged and revitalised you can feel and the better you can sleep.

And you can have a sense of what it would be like to approach a sick animal, and hovering your hands near that sick animal, and beginning to feel the sensations between your hands and that animal, and it may be like a tingling sensation, or a pressure or a warmth or a coolness, and you can have a sense of that sensation as you channel universal loving kindness into that animal, as you channel that healing energy into the energy, into the life-force of that animal.

And then you can have a sense of another situation, a totally different situation, this time you see a distressed or upset friend or family member and you instinctively go over to them and lay a hand gently on them and so softly, and as you do, you notice something wonderful begin to happen. You begin to discover that healing energy, that loving kindness flowing from your fingertips, flowing from your hand, flowing into that person. And you can notice whether you can see it happening, or whether you can just feel it happening.

And you can go into a deep and focused state of mind, almost like going into auto-pilot, where you just instinctively carry out that transmission of loving kindness. And you can be curious about what the sensation is like as you transmit that loving kindness into that friend or family member, and how you notice as it begins to take effect on them, almost as if it is contagious, spreading good, positivity and wellbeing.

And as you continue to go deeper and deeper into this guided meditation, you can honestly and fully absorb and integrate your learning about how to spread loving kindness to those that you meet. And how you can begin to increase the karma, so that the more you spread that loving kindness, the more loving kindness you get back, and this can happen instinctively.

And as you follow this meditation deeper with each breath you take you can begin to have your mind and body filled with loving kindness so that you can begin to see the world through this perspective of loving kindness, and you can be curious about how this will alter your experience of the world around you. And that loving kindness can appear to emanate from your body, and you can discover how that loving kindness emanates, whether it is in pulses or whether it is with a glow, or whether it is like electricity spreading out from your fingertips, or whether it will be like the light of your spirit.

And you can drift more comfortably as you meditate on the breath, meditate on allowing that loving kindness to spread throughout your mind, your body, your spirit and your soul. And the more you breathe as you are now, the deeper absorbed you will become. And during this meditation your mind can become free from thought, and you can enjoy freedom. And you can enjoy that freedom in a way that suits you, in a way that feels natural. And you can find yourself absorbing and learning and integrating your own self-expression of loving kindness and healing.

And meditating on your breathing can help loving kindness flow through your body, and flow out into the universe to touch on those that need it. And if there is anyone that you know that would be helped by meditating compassion and love for them and for their wellbeing you can take some time to think of them now and hold them in mind to create a connection between you and them, almost like a golden thread that can allow healing, wellbeing, compassion and loving kindness to spread from you and into them.

And your loving kindness can interact with the energy of others, it can feed in pleasure and healing and a connection with those that it touches. And get a sense of that loving kindness being transmitted into the hearts and souls of every living being. Allowing you to see and connect with the inner beauty of others, and you can see the inner beauty of other.

And there is a story about a Buddhist monk, he went to a temple and took his new expensive shoes off at the door, after he had finished praying he returned to the door only to notice his shoes were missing. The monk calmly left the temple and went home. When he arrived home he was asked where his shoes were, the monk replied that they were taken, he was asked didn't that make you angry. "No", replied the monk, "I can only apologise to the thief that I have created. Had I not worn such expensive shoes I never would have tempted a less fortunate person to feel the need to steal."

And you can discover how every unkind act leads you to feel a sense of compassion and understanding and loving kindness to others. And in a moment you can drift back to the here and now holding on to that feeling and perspective of loving kindness. And when you are ready you can open your eyes.

Gratitude meditation

Take a few moments to close your eyes and begin to focus inwardly. And as you focus inwardly you can begin to consider gratitude. And many people don't realise how much they have to be grateful for, how many things go well that they have never noticed. And this guided meditation is to help you to give gratitude for those things you are aware of, and those things you aren't aware of.

If you don't give gratitude or don't give thanks for things that go well for you, your emotional health can begin to suffer. Giving gratitude can help to lift depression and reduce anxiety and stress.

There are times things can happen that you should be grateful for, even though you don't know you should be grateful. Like someone asking to talk to you. You may be in a hurry, and in that moment you may see that person as an inconvenience, yet they may have stopped you from taking a different path, where you went out to your car a few minutes earlier and a bus drives through a puddle and splashes you ruining your smart clothes for an interview you are heading to.

Without giving gratitude people can begin to lack purpose and meaning in life, and they can struggle to get what they want in life because they are never giving back and giving thanks.

So now begin to pay attention to your hands, or perhaps pay attention to your legs, or to a sensation or feeling from within your body. And begin to pay attention to something you can focus on now. And as a part of you continues to pay attention to that sensation you can discover yourself in a garden. It can be an indoor garden, or an outdoor garden. It can be any sort of garden that you like.

And everything in that garden can represent something in your life, and you don't have to know what represents what. And begin to walk around that garden looking at different plants, and perhaps there are some animals there as well. And as you walk around you can begin to get a feeling of gratitude in your stomach, you can be curious what it feels like when you pay attention to it.

You know the feeling you get when someone gives you a gift out of love. And begin to get a sense that that garden is full of love, and that love radiates off all the plants and off of any animals that might be there. They say love is in the air. And begin to really enjoy that love. And in your mind say how grateful you are for all of those things around you, both known and unknown. Being grateful for all of those things you missed during the day. And begin to notice that with each breath out, you breathe out all the toxins that have accumulated from everyday living. You breathe out all nastiness from the day.

And begin to notice that each in-breath is breathing in love and comfort, and with each in-breath that you take that love and that comfort can begin to fill your body.

And you can have a sense of what it feels like for that love and comfort to be filling your body, what it feels like as it passes through the nose, as it enters the lungs, as it spreads around the blood and enters the cells, and in the cells it spreads right down to a genetic level.

And listening to this can create pleasurable profound effects. And as you breathe out, the out-breath can draw out any toxins, from a genetic level, from within the cells, into the blood, through the heart, into the lungs and out of the lungs via the breath.

And you can have a sense of this process, of breathing in this way, visualising this process as it happens, and you can honestly and fully give thanks on a deep level for everything throughout the day that you have received, both known and unknown. And you can continue to breathe in this way as you transfer love into every cell in your body, into every part of your genetic makeup, deep into your DNA. And each breath can carry that love deep into your heart to be passed around your body. And as you give gratitude you can increase health, harmony, happiness, wealth and success, carrying that love deep inside, and breathing out all the toxins and anything unwanted. And you don't have to know consciously what is being breathed out, and you can carry on breathing in that way, and giving gratitude for all you know and what remains unknown.

And you can listen to this guided meditation regularly to continue to effectively give gratitude and to help you continue to breathe in love, and breathe out negativity and toxins. And continue to increase health, wellbeing and happiness.

And after a few minutes of focusing on this breathing, breathing in love, and breathing out negativity, and focusing on giving gratitude you can drift back from this meditation and open the eyes. And as you go through each day you can remember to regularly acknowledge what you are grateful for. It could be being grateful for meeting someone new, it could be being grateful that a bus was arriving just as you were getting to the bus stop, or grateful for the day you have just had. And when you are ready you can drift back to the present and open your eyes.

Discover truth, enlightenment and peace

Close your eyes, and begin the process of relaxing comfortably and listen along to this guided meditation, and as you listen along you can begin to discover truth, enlightenment and peace. And you won't discover truth, enlightenment and peace in anyone else's way, you will honestly develop that discovery in your own way, and you can develop that discovery and understanding of truth, enlightenment and peace by focusing on freedom, focusing on love, having the energy to develop hope and trust with your own instinctive mind. And you can explore peace and discover creativity from within.

And the opportunity to explore the mysteries of wonder and possibilities, to evolve in your own unique way, through an exploration of consciousness and wonder, and you can wonder about the nature of reality, wonder about the possibilities of the future and the potential from within from your own personal evolution.

And as you explore your internal world through a sense of love and hope, you can trust in that exploration that you will discover a sense of self. And that exploration will take you on an unconscious evolution a chance to explore reality in new ways, a chance to master success and create new development.

And that new development can lead to a new understanding of energy, of the way energy flows around your body, and of the connection with the way energy flows around your body in all its different forms, and of information, and the way the honest expression of energy is that it is just information in many different forms.

And you can focus in your own unique way on future potentials, on movement from within, on a movement that can connect you with everyone else and with the world around you, almost like a universal movement. A movement of kindness and love that can enhance your wisdom and increase your perception and ability to change. And as you explore self-expression and wonder, you can connect in many ways to nature and to the world around you and through this deep and meaningful connection with nature and the world around you, you can achieve, meaning, you can transcend achievement, you can transcend motivation, you can be free to explore happiness.

And to really take a journey of self-discovery into your true potential, realising the vibrational energy within you and the harmony of peace and love and enlightenment of truth and hope and creativity, and all that resonates with you can begin to resonate with those around you. And you can explore the meaning of harmonic resonance, and how that leads to the discovery of the correct people in life, of people that share the same sort of values as you, of people that share the same sort of beliefs, people you can trust on your journey of love and discovery.

And you can deeply explore your perception of love, and explore how a sense of control can come from freedom, from the freedom of understanding deep mysteries that have taken an eternal journey of self-discovery to achieve that success, and to be able to then spread kindness and wonder and wisdom to others throughout your life.

And through that ability to express yourself with passion, you can begin to change the reality that you live in. By changing that perception you begin to change that reality. And you can wonder what it is you will discover from exploring love, from exploring hope, from honestly and fully exploring the mysteries of nature, of happiness, really exploring those mysteries of life.

And you can imagine a world with a universal perception, a perception where everyone sees the world through a sense of kindness, with a focus on the mysteries of life, to truly discover the wisdom of self-expression and develop an honest and full understanding of yourself, of how you personally can achieve happiness and love. Taking a journey into the exploration of possibilities and potentials. Following a path to enlightenment and wonder as you develop peace from within, and focus on your own internal development of love for yourself, for life, for nature and for those around you.

And you know love has many different meanings. And before you awaken feeling a sense of bliss, you can wonder how you can communicate change and excitement and the potential for wisdom and universal understanding. And as you have been listening to this guided meditation, some of this will have resonated with you.

And you can understand trust in your own self exploration, because your own true enlightenment will come from peace, from a sense of freedom and love, and from a sense of hope for humanity and for the world around us, and a deep harmonic resonance for those likeminded people.

And this really can be an opportunity to develop a focus on the journey of self-discovery and wonder. And that journey can take you to a place of kindness, a place of deep wisdom and change. And I know that as you listen to this you can understand what is being said and the meaning in what is being said. And you can really understand how the perception of the movement of the world around us can begin to create a universal movement, can begin to create a passion, a discovery of deep and meaningful love, of wisdom, of wonder.

To achieve success through altering the reality of the future and exploring the possibilities of the mind and the body, and developing an enlightened approach to internal understanding and hoping for the wisdom of kindness and trust.

And you can discover that the mysteries that can be found through exploration, through exploration of yourself, through exploration of the world around you, through an exploration of love, of compassion, can begin to find a way of living in harmony. And one of the most important things is to find a way of living in harmony with the world around you, with other's around you, showing a deep and meaningful understanding and respect for their perceptions, for their views.

Developing the wisdom, the understanding and the ability to attach to what is important, and to just let other things go. And as you have been following along to this you can understand what all this means, you can understand what this is all about, and it is about meeting your needs in a way that is comfortable for you, and it is about a whole lot more, and as you begin to master what has been shared here, and you begin to take the opportunity to trust what it is you can discover from within yourself, and trust that you can learn from that, and that you can take a journey into self-exploration. To begin to create wonderful feelings from within. Some people feel that happiness is something you get based on what happens to you, without realising that happiness comes from within you, that you can be in any situation and decide to be happy.

And so a part of you can explore the idea of taking a journey into self-discovery, taking a journey into self-discovery where you can discover how you can experience love, experience happiness, experience wonder, and you can experience all that from within.

And it can be as easy as just opening your eyes. And sometimes the answer to enlightenment is right under your nose. Sometimes the answer to peace, to truth and to mysteries can be contained within the heart. And you know the heart can beat out lovingly throughout your body, generating happiness and wonder and filling you with the energy to create movement and wisdom in your mind. And as you interact with others you can enhance your perception whilst you enhance their lives, through acts of kindness, and trust, and a generation of hope and discovery, focusing on creating freedom through peace and enlightenment, and discovering how you can share love and master the perception of change.

And you can create a deep belief about how to experience happiness throughout your life, and wonder, and how to change your future reality, by the development of hope and self-discovery. And before you finish exploring the possibilities of nature, the possibilities of life, the possibilities of evolution, and the mysteries around you. You can wonder how many more times you are going to listen to this and wonder whether each time you listen to this you understand it in a new and different way based on learnings you have had, or based on what your needs are at the time, and you can really be curious what it is that will make you feel good each time you listen to this.

And so you can discover the truth behind how you can create that enlightened state of peace, and develop the energy for a sense of freedom and focus, and with that development can become the discovery of love and hope, and through your creativity you can find trust and the opportunities on your journey into a mystery. And as you take a mysterious journey into an exploration of yourself you can evolve into a future with the potential for greater evolution than your old version of reality had.

And as you experience this success and begin to master the wonder of kindness, you can enhance your wisdom, and through the enhancement of your wisdom you can feel a motivation and movement and a new meaning to your perception, a new meaning to all the changes that are taking place throughout your life, a new meaning to those achievement and the communication that you have, and the deep understanding that you gain from the universal expression of nature, of discovering that everything is one. And this can give you a tremendous sense of control over various aspects of your life, and a certain kind of passion for new choices where you can feel free to experience happiness through your ability to have harmony that can really resonate with what you can discover.

And you can just take a few minutes to really understand all this on a deep and meaningful level before coming back to the here and now with a smile, knowing you can listen to this in the future as often as you would like.

Body awareness mindfulness meditation

Take a few moments to close your eyes, now this meditation is to help you to become aware of your own body, and to begin to be mindful of the information that comes in from your body and from your mind without attaching to it or being drawn into the thoughts or worries. And it is perfectly natural for your mind to wander, it is perfectly natural for worries and concerns from the day to enter your mind, the important thing is that anytime any worries or intrusive thoughts enter your mind, you allow yourself to acknowledge those thoughts and then move on by focusing on the task at hand.

And so you can take a few moments to start to focus on your breath, focusing on breathing in. And breathing out. And as you breathe in, and breathe out a few times you can begin to focus on the top of your head. And you are just focusing on allowing yourself to discover sensations and feelings that you normally overlook, in the same way that someone can put a pair of glasses on and they are aware of the glasses on their face, and after a while they stop being aware of the glasses. And to become aware of the glasses again they need to be reminded of them.

And just focus on the top of your head, and notice what feelings and sensations are there. Perhaps you can feel the hair on your head, perhaps your head is resting against something. Perhaps you can feel a warmth or a coolness, or an itchiness, or a tingling. Just notice what you can notice, and as you do this just continue to breathe in a nice deep and relaxed way, and allow your awareness to drift down to your forehead. And again notice what you can notice at your forehead, perhaps you can notice hair on your forehead, or perhaps a certain temperature.

And as you do this you are beginning to learn how to focus your attention, and beginning to learn how to focus your attention for longer and longer periods of time, which will help with learning, with concentration, with carrying out tasks. And by learning to control what you focus on, you are also learning to be able to choose what you decide to think about, which is an invaluable skill for people that perhaps find their mind worrying or have unnecessary thoughts.

So just notice what your ears feel like, allow that attention to drift to your ears, and around your jawbone and your cheeks. And what do your eyes feel like? And what does your nose feel like, and what does your mouth feel like? And just take a few breaths to allow yourself to become aware of your neck, and the top of your shoulders, aware of what your neck and the top of your shoulders feel like.

And with a few breaths allow yourself to let that focus drift down to your chest muscles, and can you feel clothes on your body, and can you feel movement with each breath, can you feel any temperature? And just allow that attention to drift down to the lower back and the stomach, being aware of the lower back and the stomach and what they feel like.

And then begin to let that awareness spread down to the lower part of your body, to your bottom, to your legs, and having an awareness perhaps of a heaviness or an immobility or of certain temperature or certain feelings in your bottom and in your legs, and also allow yourself to be aware of your arms. Do both arms feel the same, does one arm feel heavier or lighter than the other, or warmer or cooler than the other, and how about those hands and those fingers?

Really paying close attention to them, as if it is the first time you have ever discovered those hands and fingers. Looking for the most minute difference between them.

And allow that attention to go all the way down to the feet and being aware of what the feet feel like, perhaps they are resting on something, perhaps they are wearing shoes or socks, and noticing the sensations there. And then once you have become aware all the way down to the feet, start at the top of the head again, and this time imagine, as you are aware of each part of the body, that a comfortable light is filling you up from the top of the head, down to the neck, through to the shoulders and the arms, and the upper body, and the stomach, and the lower back, all the way down into your legs, and down into your feet, and really take your time to be aware of that, to allow your body to fill with a comfortable light, that can highlight the bits of your body that you have paid attention to, to make sure you have paid attention to each part of your body.

And then once you have done that and filled your whole body with a comfortable light, you can just allow your mind to focus on your breathing for a little bit and have an awareness of your whole body as a whole being, before, in your own time, drifting back to the here and now feeling so refreshed and so comfortable.

Master your imagination mindfulness meditation

Take a few moments to close your eyes and begin to listen to this mindfulness meditation to help you to master your imagination. This meditation can help you to learn to use your imagination, worrying is one example of misusing the imagination, and by learning to take control of your imagination you can then take control of worrying and other negative thoughts. Achieving success requires using your imagination for problem-solving, for rehearsing future events going as planned, and you can do this more as you take control of your imagination.

So with your eyes closed begin to get a sense of tomorrow in your mind's eye. Begin to get a sense of what you think will happen tomorrow, get a sense of things going how you want them to go, so if there is going to be any challenges or difficulties tomorrow imagine yourself going through those situations, imagine yourself dealing with any challenges or problems appropriately. Perhaps that you remains calm, perhaps that you begins to think of answers and solutions.

Whatever it is watch that you, and notice what you can see about that you, and some people say they aren't good at visualising, and if you think you are one of those people, just imagine what you think you would see.

And if anything comes up in your mind, like any thoughts of worrying, just stick with it but imagine it in a new way, imagine it as if you are imagining that you can solve the situation, and if you can't solve the situation, just imagine that it is being dealt with so that you no longer worry about it. And it doesn't matter that this is just in your imagination and not in reality, the important thing is to begin to teach your mind to think about things differently. So instead of worrying and seeing things going wrong all of the time, it is about teaching your mind to take those same things and thinking 'OK if that does happen what will I do, how will I handle that, what will happen, how will I handle the result of what happens'.

If it is worrying, for example about what others think of you or what others think of what you have done, then it is about taking that same thought, but imagining it in a different way. Imagining for example, different meaning for whatever it is that makes you think that someone would be thinking a certain thing. So it could be that you have been thinking that someone looked at you funny the other day, and you can think about what other meanings there could be for that look. Could it be that the person was just thinking about something and while they were deep in thought they looked like they were looking at you in a certain way. Could it be that they looked at you in a certain way because they have just caught a glimpse of you and they thought you were someone else that they knew so they had to take a second look to see if you were who they thought you were. So you can think of as many alternatives for their behaviour as possible.

And you can begin to learn how to think about things in a way that is resourceful and helpful to you, so that you can use your imagination and have control over your imagination instead of your imagination having control over you. And the most important thing is to begin to learn how to rehearse the future. Imagining situations that would have previously made you feel anxious or some other negative feeling, or perhaps behaviours that others do that lead to you responding in an inappropriate way, like with anger or anxiety, and you can imagine yourself responding in a more appropriate way.

And if you can't immediately imagine yourself responding in those ways, then imagine someone else in your mind in those situations, someone you know would respond in those more appropriate ways if they were in those situations. And notice what you would see, what you would hear and what you would feel as you observe that person responding in those appropriate ways. And notice what their inner dialogue is as they remain calm and relaxed or respond in their appropriate way. So take a few moments to mentally rehearse using your imagination appropriately.

(Silent for 3 minutes)

And in your own time when you feel ready to do so you can drift back to the here and now, and open your eyes. And you can listen to this as often as you need to, to practice taking control of your imagination. And you can be aware that the mind can't tell the difference between something real and something vividly imagined. So someone worrying all the time convinces the brain that this is how you should respond in the situations they are worrying about, and those situations are more likely to be full of anxiety. Someone that thinks about things going well convinces the brain that this is how things should go in those types of situations, so they have greater success, happiness and achievement.

Re-centring mindfulness meditation

Take a few moments to close your eyes and allow yourself to experience this re-centring mindfulness meditation. Now throughout the day stress and worries can begin to pile up, so it is important to re-centre your mind and body.

And one of the most effective ways to re-centre your mind and body is to sit down and close your eyes and focus on your breathing. And it is good to do this every 90-120 minutes, and this helps to keep emotion levels in check throughout the day.

So with your eyes closed, you may notice different thoughts and ideas and worries pass into your mind, and that is OK, you can just notice those thoughts and ideas and worries, and acknowledge them and then you can just let them go and focus your attention back to your breathing.

And you can focus on your breathing, and you can focus on breathing from the stomach so that the stomach moves in and out with each breath, so that you are filling your lungs from the top of your lungs all the way down to the bottom of your lungs, and when you exhale you can exhale fully, so that you exhale all of the air that is in your lungs, so that you are taking very long breaths.

And as you do it can help to breathe through the nose or mouth, whichever is most comfortable for you, and you can notice the feelings associated with each breath. And if your mind wanders to different thoughts and ideas, there is no need to tell yourself off about it or judge yourself about it, it is perfectly natural, instead you can just bring your attention back to your breathing, back to your stomach and to the movement of your stomach.

So take time to focus on your breathing, it could be on the movement of the stomach with each breath, or the movement of other muscles, perhaps the muscles around the sides, or the chest muscles. It could be focusing on the movement of the nostrils or the mouth as you breathe in and out. It could be focusing on the temperature or the feeling of each breath as it goes in and out of your mouth or nose and as the air travels down your windpipe.

And you can take a few moments of peace and quiet to focus on breathing in and out, allowing all of your attention to be focused on each breath that you take, as if you can see in your mind's eye each breath going in and out, whilst at the same time you can feel each breath coming in and going out. And you can hear each breath going in and going out. And you can take a minute to focus on that now.

(Silent for 1 minute)

And with practice you can master this mindfulness re-centring meditation, and with practice you can extend the time you focus on breathing in and breathing out, and as you improve you can extend the period of time you can hold this focus for three minutes, for five minutes or even for ten minutes, without the need for this guided meditation, focusing on breathing in and breathing out. Re-centring the mind and body, and anytime the mind wanders, with practice you will be able to comfortably bring the mind back to the breath.

And as you begin to master this technique you will begin to be calmer throughout the day, you will begin to improve your ability to focus your attention on what you want to focus on, and will begin to improve being able to control your attention, and to manage stressful situations, and to think clearer. And you will notice many other benefits from practicing and mastering re-centring mindfulness meditation.

And you can now take a few moments to comfortably drift back to the here and now and open your eyes.